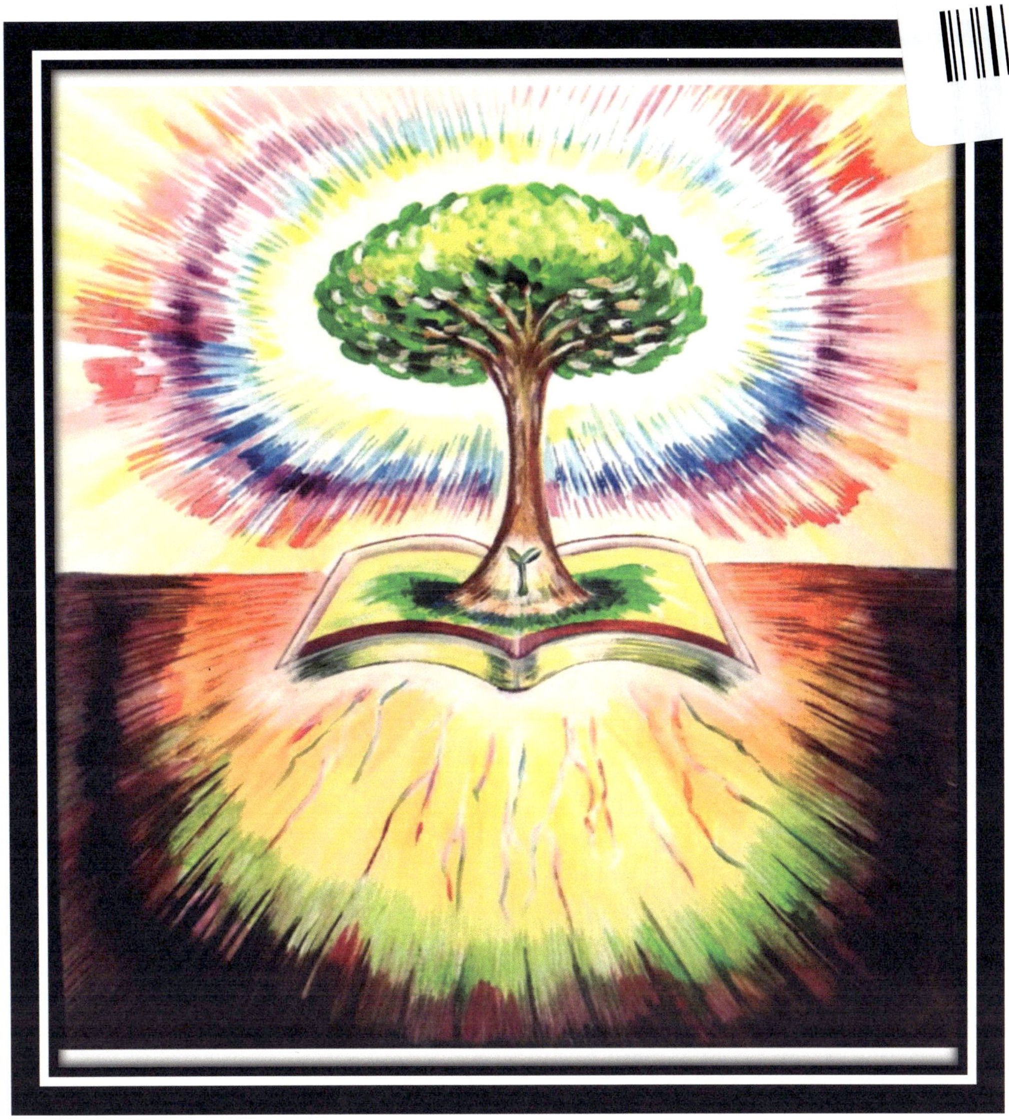

HEART OF A DOULA, BIRTHING A VISION

Jessica LaFavor

Published by:
R.H. Publishing
Dallas, TX. 75240

ISBN#978-1-960494-08-5

Cover illustration by Yoon Soo Nam

ACKNOWLEDGMENTS

To my mother Rose, your continued support, prayer, and encouragement have always given me the motivation I needed to walk the path that I was called to in my life. The example of sacrifice, devotion, and strength you have shown, has been a testimony of God's grace and your servant's heart. For this, I will always be grateful. I will forever treasure the embracing moments that you and I have shared on this journey together—you are truly a woman of strength! The legacy of family and the ancestorial heritage of native tradition has been a guiding light.

To my three children, Samuel, Christine, and Noah. Each of your births was a total miracle and you have been more of a gift to me than you will ever know. It is a blessing to be your mother and a joy to see God's purpose fulfilled in your life. My prayer for each of you is this, that you may live a life dedicated to being healthy, growing, and full of love for generations to come! For Abby and Jess, my wonderful daughters-in-love, you are such blessings to our family.

For both of my sisters, I would not be the woman I am today if it were not for the specific influences that each of you brought into my life. Jennifer, I will never forget the honor that it was to be a part of your journey, as we both entered motherhood. This was the first inspiration that eventually led me to become a doula! Joanna, the friendship, and unity we share have made this work complete, you are so treasured. Thank you for believing in me. I know that we both have co-labored together through many trials to come to this place of purpose!

This labor of love was made possible through much prayer and insight from the entire Grateful Life Ministries team and Church! Thank you for helping me fulfill my vision! A special thanks go out to Robert and Jen, Judi, AmyJo, Sheri, Laura, Steph, Sara, Jill, Julie, Nancy, Carol and to my publisher, and friend Polly. To Embery for bringing enlightenment to my heart and giving me a new perspective on my work, my purpose, and who I am. I appreciate all the beautiful families whom I held sacred space with as they had their babies. Finally, I cannot adequately express the gratitude I have to God for bringing me from death to life, being my healer and giving me the creativity and power that I have experienced throughout this amazing journey!

TABLE OF CONTENTS

INTRODUCTION

The daughter of a lion is also a lion—African Proverb. This speaks to our identity in the kingdom of God, royalty as co-heirs with Christ, and destiny as women of strength; those who are charged with the honor of servanthood and mentorship. Weren't women always in attendance at births traditionally? Yes, they were … and they should be! Long before I was a doula, I had the honor of entering motherhood with my sister Jennifer. My niece, Maricella, was born 8 days after my son, Samuel, and this experience would be the inspiration for my future doula career. My sister had a very difficult pregnancy and we both experienced traumatic childbirth experiences. The journey we had throughout the postpartum period and into parenting solidified the importance of having support, education, advocacy, and presence during pregnancy, labor, delivery, and the days following.

Years later my youngest sister Joann and I lived in separate states but had a common vision to save lives through doula care. The main reasons women have abortions are that they feel alone, unsupported, and afraid. We each had a doula business, hers called *Miracle of Life* and mine called *Embracing Moments*. We recognized the parallel that there was in physical and spiritual new life. We formed a non-profit called Embracing Miracles to be a resource for those pursuing wholeness. We have learned together what it means to be, women of strength instead of strong women. The passing down of ancient wisdom is essential to mothers, wives, sisters, daughters, and all women. This creates community, support, and courage.

One thing we focus on is spiritual mentorship for women in our communities and around the world! We want you to experience empowerment and encouragement that will change your life and equip you to walk in victory. At no other time in history has it been so crucial that women and families have the support necessary to choose life! As we provide the essential components of information and application to those who have the heart to serve all women and especially those experiencing unplanned pregnancy, lives will be saved! Not only that, but we need to remember the importance of storytelling and releasing past pain. As a woman living in long-term term recovery, I have been in the rooms of AA and NA as well as *Celebrate Recovery* where we used the word grateful to share our testimony…learned to have an attitude of gratitude and found out that we never walk alone. These are things that help us heal.

I was very honored to receive my first DONA birth doula training from Gail Tully (Spinning Babies) in 2007 and was certified in 2010. I was overcome by the powerful validation I felt throughout the weekend that this is not something I did, but who I was! I had been a part of the birth stories of all my nieces and nephews in either prayer or presence. The first birth I attended after my training was for Bruce and Rebecca Williams. The labor of their son Aaron was 22 ½ hours long and I remember when I got home thinking this was exactly where I belonged. As has been the case with so many families, I was invited back for another birth when they had their daughter Naomi.

I became a pastor in 2011 and I had the vision to start Grateful Life Ministries in 2012. The outline for what would become the "Heart of a Doula, Birthing a Vision" workshop came to me in a matter of 20 minutes, it took the next 4 years to write the rest of the content. During this journey, I recalled the many conversations and prayer I had with Nancy, Nate, Dale, Melodie, and Shay at the Rochester Outreach Center. It was here, that *Grateful Life* found its heart. Later as I served in the church, my shepherding gift was supported by Steph, Johann, and Deb. God met me in a powerful way during this time and showed me His compassion and guidance. Isaiah 40:11 says, "He will tend his flock like a shepherd; he will gather the lambs in his arms; he will carry them in his bosom, and gently lead those that are with young."

Our mission as doulas is love at birth, love for life—walking alongside those on the journey of new life, providing co-laboring birth and postpartum support physically and spiritually. Our goal is to specialize in Christian doula training to mentor women in becoming professional doulas, cultivate a community resource, the *Grateful Life Doula Collective*, and provide affordable childbirth education, doula care, and trauma healing for families. We want to see the next generation rise as "ministry doulas"—those who know how to become co-laborers in their own communities. I knew it was God's plan and will for my life to equip, empower, and encourage people to be spiritually healthy, growing, and full of love—not only for one another but for themselves, as well.

We do this in four ways:

1.) Seminars—education
2.) Workshop—training
3.) Resources—community
4.) Retreats—healing

CHAPTER 1

WHAT IS THE ROLE OF A DOULA

As doulas, it is important to recognize our role as we participate in the process of walking alongside those on the journey of new life. It is an honor to be a part of such an intimate moment with others. We must remember to uphold the standard of what it means to be of service as we continue the work we have been called to do. Having a grateful life comes from knowing the love and light of God and letting your light shine on others. It means creating a safe place of hospitality and warmth. We are professional yet know how to show compassion.

Having a teachable spirit is just as important as being an expert in your field and sharing your knowledge with others. When we learn, we can grow. Growth leads to new experiences and the illumination of our perspective. Our desire is to understand that we have been a part of a system that uses institutional power to determine what is best for others when it comes to their birth experience and to be aware of the privilege, we may be exerting in our doula practice. All nations are from one blood (Acts 17:26), realizing our humanity is foundational in providing equitable care, education, support, and advocacy.

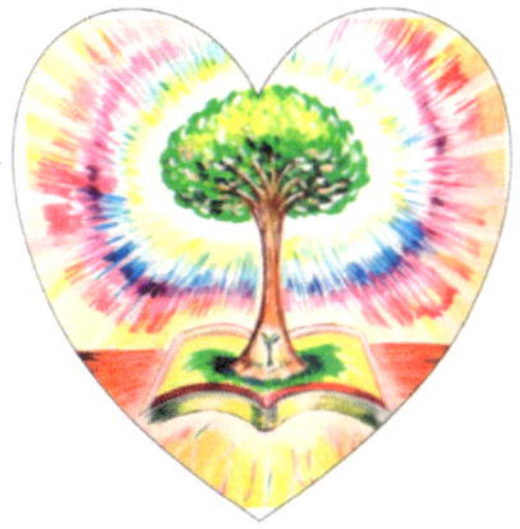

Grateful Life Ministries- Love at Birth, Love for Life!

Scope of Practice: Ethics/Action

- Professional values and personal commitment
- Professional skills and abilities
- Professional knowledge and understanding
- Providing compassion within pre-established boundaries
- Reflection for other's potential
- Nurturing Leadership

Code of Honor for DOULAS

Devotion toward new life

Observant as a co-laborers

Unifying as a whole team

Leadership in community

Assertive in difficult moments

Strength to empower others

WHAT IS A DOULA?

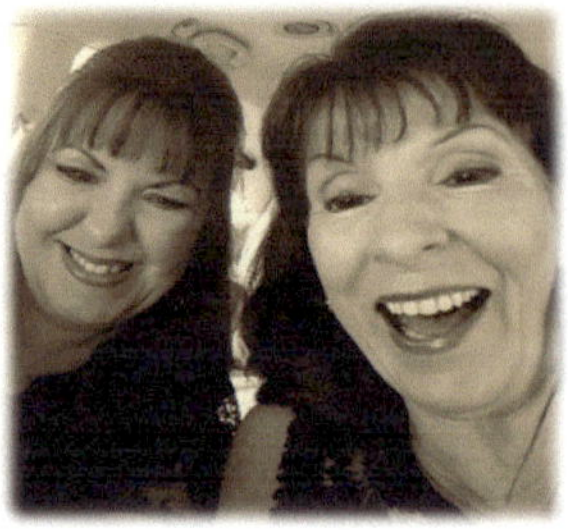

My mother Rose has always been known for her serving heart.

The word "doula" comes from the ancient Greek meaning, "**a woman who serves**." A doula provides continuous physical, emotional, informational, and [spiritual] support to the mother before, during, and after the birth. She provides emotional and practical support during the postpartum period after delivery. In the case of a *ministry doula*, she is present in the time of transition and provides mentorship, resources, and prayer.

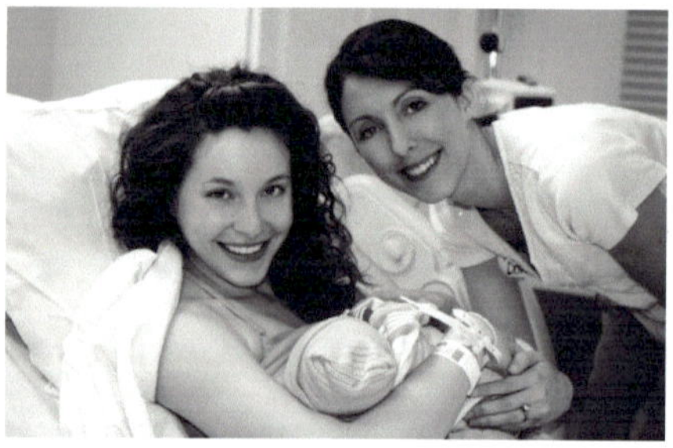

Joanna Pixley providing postpartum doula care after labor and delivery.

WHY BE A DOULA?

When you love a mother at the birth of her child, she is supported in loving her baby as well as herself. When you love a baby at birth, it can last a lifetime. Not only do we have love for birth, but we also have love for life itself. God being the Creator, establishes life; both physically and spiritually- we are His partners. Women are empowered by walking together. To be a Grateful Life doula is to be a servant whether in physical delivery or spiritual discipleship.

As a woman, there is nothing more precious than being invited into a miracle. The miracle of life is the heartbeat of God. Embracing moments like this is truly an honor. To fulfill the purpose and calling of a doula, one must learn to be a woman of strength; this means being one who shares their wisdom and experience with other women to bring healing. Grateful Life Ministries LLC provides a way for this to happen through partnerships like the one with Embracing Miracles, a non-profit organization dedicated to giving resources to those on the journey of wholeness.

Abortion is predominate in our society because many women even in the church feel afraid, alone, and unsupported… but what if they did not have to? What if *Doulas* were there to show compassion? What if **you** were there, so they were not alone? To be a co-laborer in your own community provides a valuable resource and a place of safety for women and families. Jesus said to serve one another, this is just one way. Do you have the heart of a doula?

Embracing Miracles: Heart of a Doula- 50 min. video Seminar

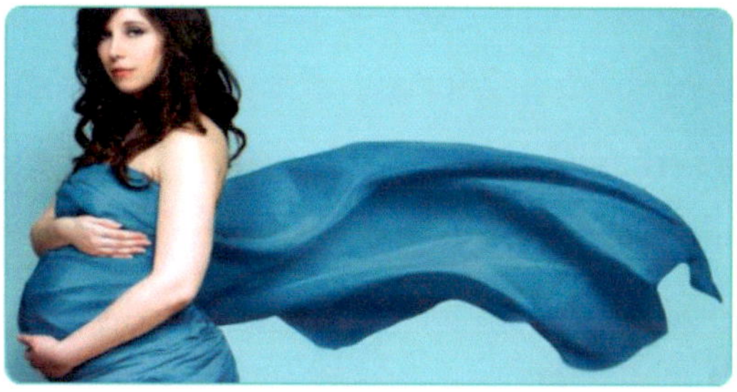

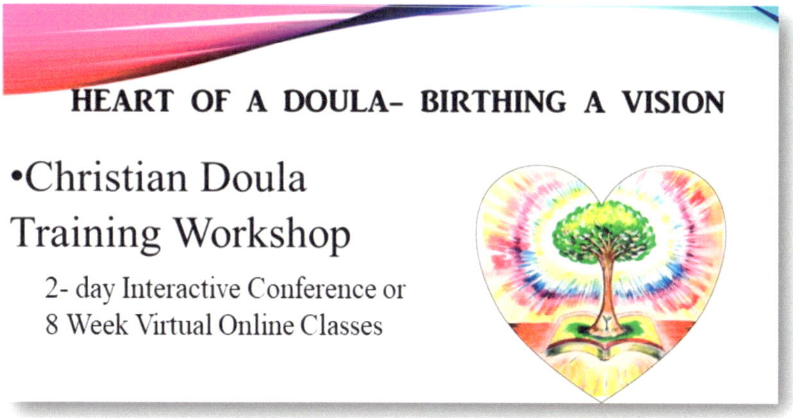

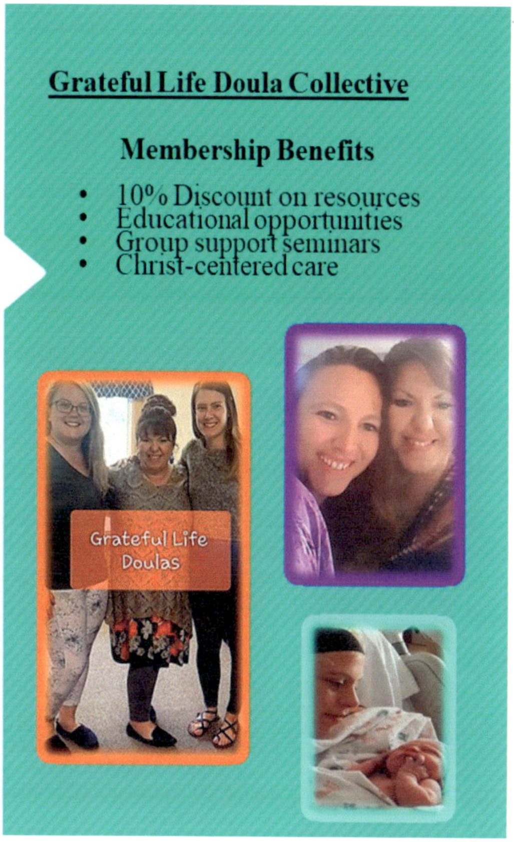

WHAT DOES A DOULA DO?

- A doula understands the physiology of birth and the emotional needs of a woman in labor. She feels the energy of the birth space and responds with observation first.
- She is there to assist the woman in preparing for and carrying out her plans for childbirth. This may include Grateful Life Childbirth Education or trauma healing.
- She stays with the woman throughout the labor providing spiritual and emotional support, physical comfort measures, and information she needs to make informed decisions. In my practice, I have back-up and partner doulas or apprentices too.
- She communicates with the laboring woman, her partner, and her clinical care providers. Though she is an advocate, she does not speak for her client or the family.
- She perceives her role as a nurturing and helpful assistant for the best birth experience possible. Being trauma informed helps the doula to provide competent care.
- She allows the woman's partner to participate at their comfort level.

The day I found out I was expecting was a precious moment in my life! My first son Samuel, which means: "One heard or asked of God", was a complete miracle since doctors had told me I would probably not be able to have children because of my two heart surgeries. It was a traumatic birth ending in a cesarean. I hemorrhaged and had to have two blood transfusions to save my life and it was a long recovery, but there was much to be thankful for… I was a mother. I had 2 miscarriages and then got pregnant with Christine; she is my rainbow baby! She was named after my mother's mother who died before I was born meaning "Anointed follower of Christ". Christine was diagnosed at 2 years old with Autism, but she would not be defined by labels or limitations! (That's a story for another book). Then, I was pregnant with baby #3.
The morning of my ultrasound my devotion was about the dove that was sent out after the flood and how there was nowhere for her to land, so she came back to Noah, which means: "One who gives rest". That is exactly how I felt; I had a 4yr.old who was totally full blast ahead, a 10-month-old I was still nursing full time, and almost 6 months pregnant. We found out we were having a son that morning and the Lord showed me how he was a symbol of Restoration. There is a purpose for every child!

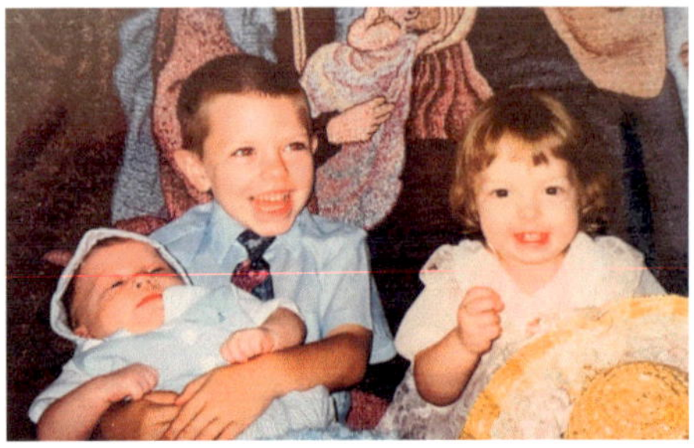

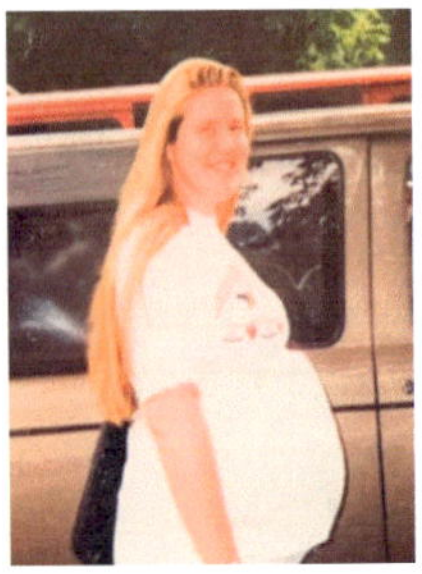

The second birth I ever attended was for my friend Laura. We met in high school, were the maids of honor at each other's weddings, and attended the birth of our firstborn! In preparation for her daughter Hannah's arrival, we prayed, read lots of material on pregnancy, and childbirth as well as practiced relaxation techniques. She had a beautiful 5-hour first-time labor and natural delivery. Even though our children are grown now, we cherish our friendship.

Women have complex needs during pregnancy, childbirth and the weeks that follow.
In addition to medical care and the support of their companions, women need consistent, continuous reassurance, comfort, encouragement, and respect. Each woman has different needs because of their individual situation. The American Congress of Obstetricians and Gynecologists, the Society of Obstetricians and Gynecologists of Canada and the World Health Organization all have recognized the benefits of doula care around the world.

CHAPTER 2

WHY HAVE A DOULA?

Research shows parents who receive support can:

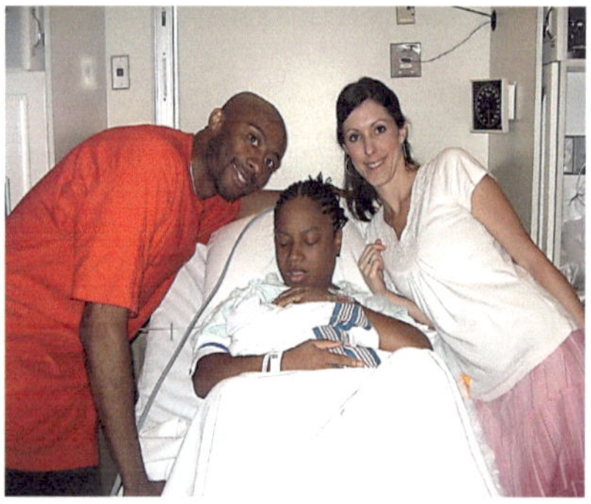

Reducing racial birth disparities among families of color is a priority for us.

- Feel more secure and cared for
- Are more successful in adapting to new family dynamics
- Have greater success with breastfeeding
- Have greater self-confidence
- Have less postpartum depression
- Have lower incidence of abuse

Clinical studies show many advantages to having a doula's presence at birth:

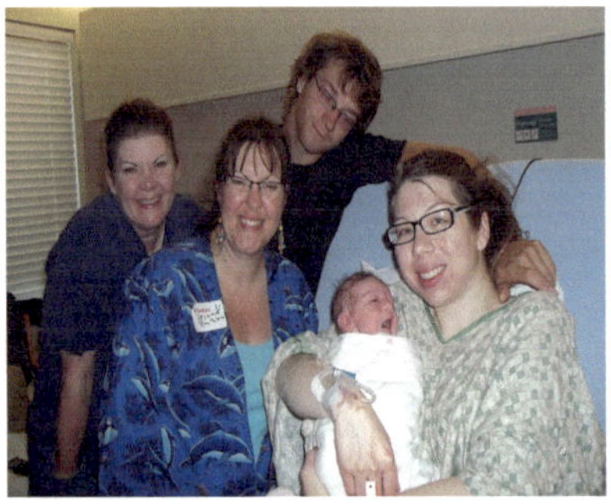

Jessica providing birth support and doula care for Alyssa and Aaron with Grandmother Laurie present for this joyful occasion.

- Result in shorter labors with fewer complications.
- Reduces negative feelings about the birth.
- Reduces the need for Pitocin (a labor-inducing drug), forceps, or vacuum extraction and cesareans.
- Reduces the mother's request for pain medication and/or epidurals.
- Women have a higher chance of a VBAC after a cesarean with a doula.
- Partners tend to stay more connected… many partners are eager to be involved during labor and birth.

HOW DOES HAVING A DOULA MAKE A DIFFERENCE?

Our walk with you is a journey, not an event. We share life together!

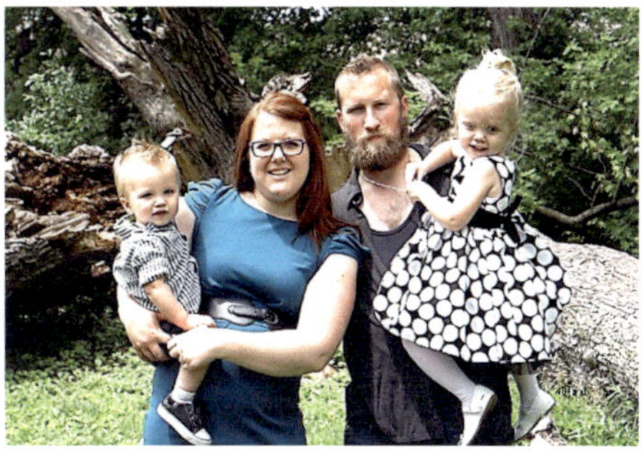

Mark and Sara Eidem with their daughter Elizabeth and son Zander.

Sara— "It was good to have someone there who was so calm and comforting. You knew just what I needed, and the lavender oil was wonderful!"

Mark—"You helped remember what was important in the moment. I think everyone should have a Doula! You even remembered food for me, thanks."

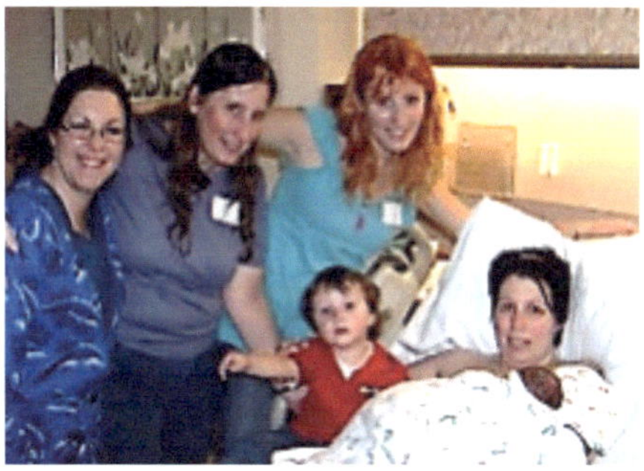

Amanda—"It was the constant assurance, praise, and prayer. Thank you for supporting me in having my son in the room when his little sister was born. I really wanted to have a natural childbirth and with your help, *I did it!*"

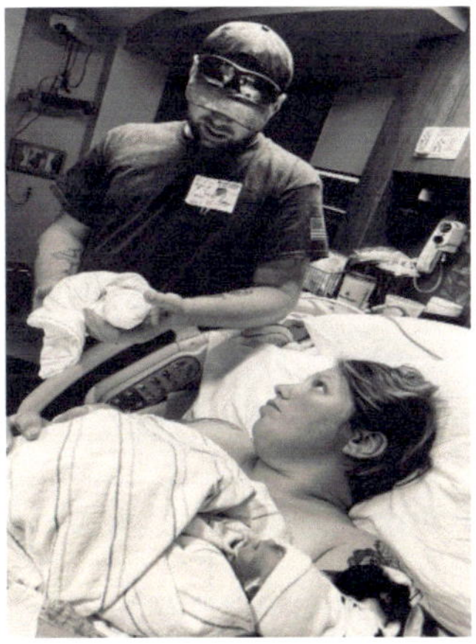

Amanda Eidem gave birth to her beautiful daughter Elvira with her mother Jill and sister Katie in the room. It was also crucial for her to have her son Logan be there to witness his siters birth. (Above)

Over a decade later, Jessica was there to bring comfort and support to Amanda and her husband Levi who lost identical triplet daughters: Faith, Lyda and Mable (May 26, 2021).

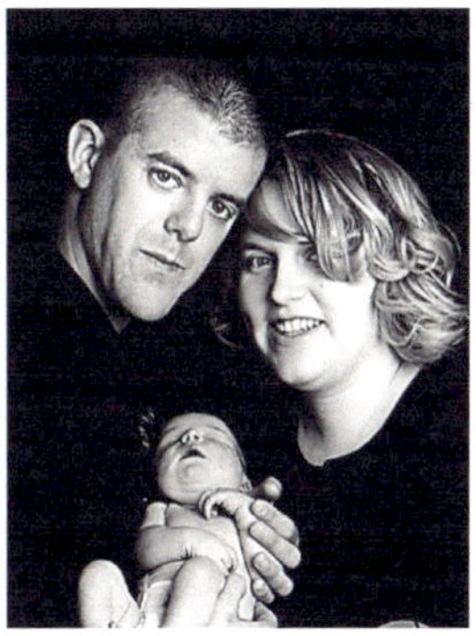

As Bryan and Carrie Casey prepared for a military tour of duty, they scheduled an induction. however, Pitocin caused low blood pressure, so they welcomed their son via caesarean.

Bryan & Carrie—"You were there for us during Bryan's mobilization just before he was deployed to Iraq; we were so grateful for all your support!"

WIFE OF A SOLDIER (CARRIE AND BRYAN'S STORY)

"With our firstborn, my husband was deploying to Afghanistan (his 3rd deployment with the army but my first). I don't know how we would have made it through without, first and foremost, God, but also the amazing support that He gave us in our angel and doula, Jessica LaFavor. As a first-time mom, I was already a big ball of nerves, then add in my husband leaving for mobilization. Let's just say— "not a fun situation." Jessica was incredibly informative every step of the way and then supported every decision we made like it was her own. She wasn't there to make decisions for us or to bully us into what was a "perfect birth" (as if there is such a thing), but she was a pillar of support and confidence, helping us remember that what we were aiming for was simply "happy & healthy" and nothing more.

In the end, our particular story ended with my husband flying in from his mobilization site in Texas about an hour before the beginning of our induction, followed by a non-emergency C-section. This meant that Jessica could not continue to be at my side for the surgery (since my husband had made it back in time for the induction—my #1 choice at the birth was him). Scared because I had never had ANY surgery before (not even tonsils or wisdom teeth), Jessica reiterated what the doctors had told us and prayed with us. After choosing the C-section, she supported us and calmed my nerves.

Then, through tears, I asked her to sit with my parents in the waiting room. She said, "I'm not going home until I get to see this baby!" My mom was so thankful to have an experienced hand to hold and shoulder to lean on. My parents are to this day so thankful for her presence that day.

The day I went home from the hospital, my husband deployed, leaving me to figure out this whole baby thing on my own, including not making enough milk for a hungry "Casey" boy and the guilt that subsequently fell. Jessica checked in on me often to offer support (and not just "How's the baby?" support) and a listening ear.

I've had two babies since then: a planned C-section (which Jessica was on-call for) and another non-emergency C-section (which 3 boys in 3 years was by this point in time, old hat). Through it all, there are 3 things I am THEE most thankful for:

1—Jessica with my mom during the first surgery—seriously they should have a "momma of the baby momma doula."

2—Jessica's encouragement through the difficult parts of the first year.

3—(and the one that still makes me tear up) Jessica helping me emphasize to the doctors and nurses (and my husband) the importance of my husband in the birth.

Jessica kept saying, "I'm not here to take the place of your loved ones. I'm here to provide experienced support," which I didn't completely understand until I was in full induced labor and my husband (who went to all the classes with me) was saying, "What can I do?" He was completely frozen, while I was hunched over a ball, doing everything I could do to not scream and cry.

Even through the C-section (of 1 & 3), he was asked by the surgical team, "Ok, Daddy, want to cut the cord?" (On #2 he decided to watch the procedure. He got woozy and had to sit—ha, soldier boy!)

I am so thankful for our friendship with Jessica! God has blessed our family in more ways than we can count through her!"

Carrie Casey

CHAPTER 3

THE PURPOSE AND VALUE OF LABOR SUPPORT

A doula's role is that of service to another woman during childbirth. It is a combined support and comfort presence and encouragement. A doula is a primary source of emotional and physical care. She has knowledge of a woman's anatomy and the stages of labor. The doula is someone who will remain throughout the entire church childbirth process and help with relaxation techniques, encouraging words, and be helpful in getting the mother started with feeding the baby. She will also give support to a woman's partner and be available to offer information and suggestions. A doula will help women discover their strengths and be confident in their own ability. She is a gentle light to labor with… my role as a doula was first discovered long before I knew the term. I have assisted with many pregnant and laboring women in their journey towards delivery. I find my role a joyful privilege in helping to bring forth new life.

The benefits of having support and labor to the mother and her family are tremendous. There are statistical findings such as those published in the donor position paper the birth doula's contribution to modern maternity care. These results showed the benefits included decrease in cesarean delivery medications emotional stress on mothers,' vacuum or forceps, increased satisfaction for birth experience and higher Apgar scores at 5 minutes.

Then there is the factor of how partners can be more a part of the whole process when they know labor support is available for the woman. Many partners are empowered to take an active role by pouring in the love they share with each other and their baby. They are also free to take care of themselves make decisions and be a good source of encouragement. Also, women feel a higher degree of control self-esteem and success with a doula who builds upon the foundation of generations of motherhood.

Another point of value is maternal bonding when a doula is present, she can help with nursing and take care of the details that allow a mother to focus on her baby. This bond in an intimate part of how a person perceives themselves for the rest of their lives. When care is given, it strengthens the family. My responsibilities as a doula can range in variabilities. Anything from physical comforts such as aromatherapy or massage counterpressure for back pain relaxation techniques soft touch encouraging words having understanding. It can also be advised throughout pregnancy labor and birth as well as to help. Julie is a word that defines what compassionate womanhood is all about we know each other's others experience and share the common thread of life-giving power.

A doula is one who will promote the growth and health of society as a whole by impacting an individual. As stated by the standards of practice through DONA International a doula's scope of practice is limited to mainly physical and emotional support, in my case, I also add a spiritual component. She is there to provide non-medical assistance so she will not offer prescriptions or examinations. In addition, a doula may make referrals and resources in the community available to our clients. My commitment is to uphold a professional code of ethics with my colleague's clients and medical staff and community. I will improve upon my knowledge and learn from my experiences. The basic responsibility of a doula is that of service with integrity. The purpose of providing labor support is simply because it's necessary. Women need other women to share in this most natural purpose of childbearing to gain knowledge asked for guidance be vulnerable in complete confidence and be empowered in motherhood. A lifetime of emotions will be filled through those memories of her child being born. It is a deep honor to be asked to be a part of such a powerful moment- this is how we have the heart of a doula.

Ashley is a woman living in long term recovery. She was in Teen Challenge during her pregnancy and transferred to transitional housing right before the birth of her son. Prenatal and birth support is essential to build a solid foundation for the future!

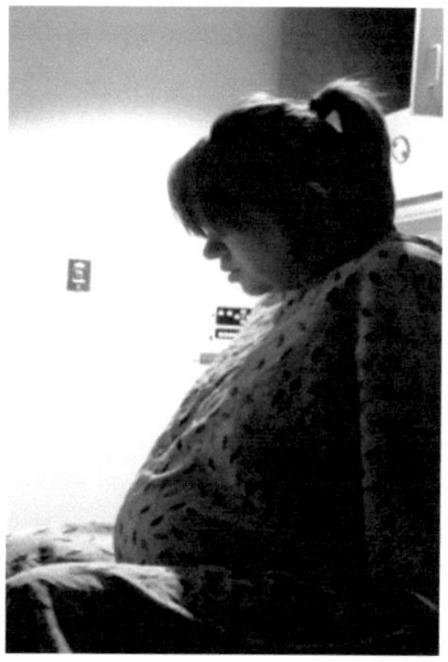

THE UNPLANNED DOULA (AMANDA AND ANDREW'S STORY)

"My two natural, unmedicated births have been almost as different as night and day. When I was birthing my first daughter, I was very fearful and struggled with panic throughout most of my labor and delivery. Unfortunately, three other women were giving birth in the hospital at the same time as me, and my midwife was unable to do much besides peak into my room occasionally. My nurse, bless her, was too encumbered by the regulations of the hospital to be of any service to me until after my daughter was born. She would only occasionally tell me to quiet down and calm down, and she only touched me to administer the fetal monitoring.

Bethany shot out of my body and ended up tearing me up extensively. I endured two hours of surgery almost immediately after she was born. She was (and sometimes still is) an incredibly high-needs baby. She was consistently fussy unless I let her nurse literally 24/7. As a result of that and stress, I didn't have an adequate milk supply, and she struggled to grow until she was 5 months old, and I was able to start her on cereal mixed with formula. I really believe my labor and delivery affected her temperament. My entire birthing experience with her was one that made me shudder and recoil at the thought of going through that again. When I found out I was pregnant with Kathryn a year and a half later, I knew I had to do something different. I knew that for me to make it through this birth more successfully, I needed my mother and my doula, Jessica, as well as my husband present. My husband was timid at the thought of other people being present at the birth, so I began talking about having Mom and Jessica there early on in my pregnancy, so he would have time to get used to the idea. I needed to tactfully approach it because I didn't want him to feel like his support was inadequate for me. I tried to explain that a doula would be a support for both of us and would not take his place. We reached the end of my pregnancy undecided.

My labor with Kathryn was very different from Bethany's, and I was unsure if I was in labor or not and what I should do. I was able to call Jessica in the middle of the night and get encouragement and advice from her. Later the next morning, my mom came and sat with me to help keep me calm because I had told my husband to go to work since I was unsure if I was really in labor or not. Jessica kept checking in by phone, and by the afternoon when my contractions finally started picking up in pace, she "stopped by."

She was a great support in reminding me to breathe and to relax between contractions. It was almost time for Andrew to get home from work so she had me tell him to pick up food for himself because she thought we would be heading to the hospital soon. He made it home, had time to scarf down a sandwich and we were off to the hospital. In triage, while we were waiting for the birthing room with the tub, Jessica showed Andrew a way to massage my back to ease the pain, and she pulled out some essential oils for a little aromatherapy. I went into the tub immediately when we were ushered into my room. Jessica and Andrew sat by me, encouraging me and helping me to stay calm and controlled. They took turns massaging my back. After an hour of relaxing in the tub, I rotated to the birthing ball where I entered my final stage of labor. Jessica just happened to have some comforting classical music available to play when I requested it.

The best part of my labor was when I began to panic because of the pain, and suddenly, I had three pairs of hands holding me down in a very comforting support while Andrew, my mom, and Jessica all started to pray out loud for me. How I needed that! When I was ready to push, I sat on the birthing chair and Jessica and Andrew stood next to me to support my body while my nurse and midwife, who had mostly just been watching my labor, prepared for the baby. I was overjoyed to have these three loved people witness sweet little Kathryn's birth. She is a very content, happy child, which I contribute in part to the fact that her birth was not as traumatic for me as her older sister's birth was. Afterwards, I asked my husband if he minded that mom and Jessica ended up staying in the room with us, and he confessed that it really took the pressure off of him, and he was happy that Jessica was there and was so prepared for every need we had. He said he didn't really understand what a doula was for beforehand, but he was really grateful we ended up with one. So am I! I can't even remember all the things Jessica did to help, but I know it would not have been as good of an experience without her.

Amanda Waltson

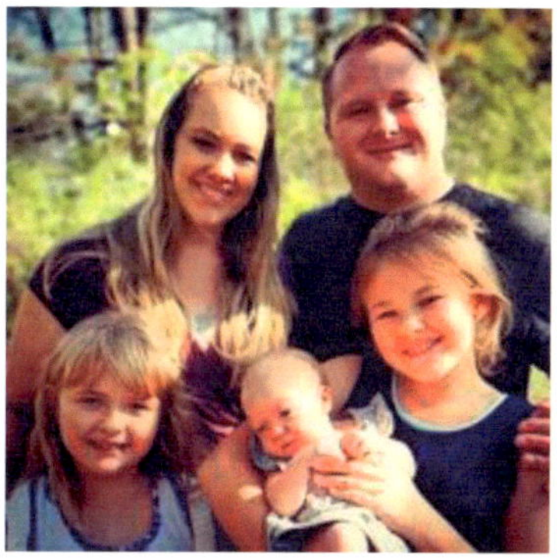

THE ROLE AND SCOPE OF BIRTH DOULA PRACTICE

The concept of labor support or having access to a birth doula is well-documented from ancient art to present-day evidence-based research. Additionally, labor doulas provide the emotional, educational, and spiritual support that has shown to make significant positive differences in labor and birth outcomes. The home birth community as well as hospitals recognize the vital role that birth doulas play as a member of the maternity health care team. A birth doula is someone who provides physical, emotional, and informational support to women during the birth process. The term 'doula' (pronounced DOOlah) is derived from a Greek term meaning female servant. Doulas are trained professionals who recognize that the right kind of support is an essential key to a positive birth experience. They support the physical and emotional needs of women in labor. They provide information that helps the woman make informed decisions with her healthcare providers. In addition, doulas offer guidance and community resources to families regarding self-care, lactation, and other issues pertinent to healthy parenting through the first six weeks postpartum. A doula provides emotional, educational, and physical support.

In contrast to the doula's role, a labor and delivery nurse tends to the clinical needs of the laboring woman in a hospital or birth center. A nurse who studies further to become a Certified Nurse Midwife can deliver babies and prescribe medicine. A monitrice, who may or may not be a nurse or a midwife, has received training in clinical skills related to birth, such as checking fetal heart tones, maternal blood pressure, and cervical change. Benefits of Birth Doula Care Statistical data from one of the largest study reviews (Hodnet, et al, 2012) demonstrates the following benefits for women who have labor support and women who do not.

Women who do have labor support are:

- 28% less likely to have a cesarean section.
- 31% less likely to use synthetic oxytocin to speed up labor.
- 9% less likely to use any pain medication.
- 34% less likely to rate their childbirth experience negatively.

Over twenty years of research and a multi-clinical trial study (Klaus, et al, 2002) show that doulas can have a significant impact on the birth process. It is important to point out, however, that if a birthing facility has taken steps to reduce the cesarean section rate, then the first percentage value may not be precise.

 50% reduction in the cesarean rate

 25% shorter labor 60% reduction in epidural requests

 40% reduction in oxytocin (Pitocin) use

 30% reduction in analgesia use

 40% reduction in forceps delivery

Scope of Doula Practice Prior to birth, a doula provides information to her clients about the birth process in general, a variety of comfort measures and coping skills, and common procedures. The doula should offer evidence-based information in a manner as unbiased as possible. Referring the client to reliable sources so that she can make her own decisions imparts confidence that she can draw upon during labor. A doula provides continuous care.

She should have arrangements to provide for her client's care in case she is unable to attend the birth. A doula provides culturally appropriate emotional support to the laboring woman, helping her to cope with labor in her own way. The doula, as a servant, lays aside any preconceived ideas she may have and supports the mother in the way that the mother chooses to labor. A doula also supports the father and others who are present, helping them to participate in the birth experience to the extent that they are comfortable. A doula physically supports the mother in a variety of ways. She will suggest alternative positions for the mother, remind her to maintain her fluid intake, make sure she goes to the bathroom frequently, or offer the use of heat/cold therapy for stress and pain relief. A doula may help with coping skills such as breathing techniques, relaxing touch or visualization. She may suggest dimming the lights or playing music —whatever creates a soothing environment for the mother.

There is a misconception that doulas only provide care for those interested in natural childbirth/unmedicated births. Doulas provide care for women with and without pain medication, unaccompanied teen mothers, women who have little or no social support, women who have disabilities, women who have cesarean sections … or women who are planning a TOLAC (trial of labor after cesarean) or VBAC (vaginal birth after cesarean). Since the core of the doula's belief is to make this the very best birth experience for a woman, the doula can be a benefit regardless of the circumstances surrounding a birth. A doula does not give medical advice or perform any medical tasks. While it is beneficial for a doula to be knowledgeable about medical procedures, her job is not to make decisions for the client. She may describe a procedure, explain why it is done, clarify the procedure's risks and benefits, and explain any alternatives (Gentry, et al, 2010).

In many cases, when clients have questions about medical issues, the doula can consider it an opportunity to facilitate communication between the client and her caregivers. When the woman and her family speak directly with her healthcare providers, it reduces risk of miscommunication and increases shared decision making. Doulas do not contradict health care providers… Entering an adversarial relationship with that provider undermines the woman's confidence in her provider and in her ability to make her own choices (ICEA, 2013).
An adversarial relationship may also affect not only her credibility in the community, but that of her doula colleagues.

It is a doula's responsibility to maintain professional relationships with others caring for the mother, such as her family, as well as with her healthcare providers. A doula protects the privacy of her clients. Per HIPAA, no personal health information (PHI) should be shared unless the client has given her express consent (Stevens, et al, 2011). Doulas provide a bridge in the maternity care gap. Continuous labor support has been shown to have positive pregnancy outcome benefits, including improved satisfaction with the birth and a rise in self-esteem of the mother. This could positively impact the mother-baby relationship in the postpartum period as well as breastfeeding initiation and continuance (Gruber, et al, 2013; Hodnet, et al, 2012; Klaus, et al, 2002). Doula care should be available to every woman who needs or wants continuous labor support.

THE SANCTITY OF LIFE

The value of human life that God places on His most precious creation is shown in the way that He deals with the end of that life, which is death. The cause of a human being's death is of great interest to God as Creator. He made people in His own image and incorporates a justice system to maintain the sanctity of life. In God's sight there is a clear distinction between intentional murder and involuntary manslaughter. The difference in these two motives make the determination for what kind of justice should be served to the perpetrator. In this research paper, several different types of death will be looked at to see the various responses that God has to life being taken. It will also show how different people groups have dealt with the value of human life in their own cultures. In the commentary of the Old Testament book of Numbers by author Gordon Wenham (2008), God institutes cities of "Refuge" for those who have killed someone. This is to provide a place of safety from the "Avenger of Blood" or "Kinsman Redeemer" who would otherwise have the legal right to execute the guilty party. This person may dwell in the city until a trial to determine the circumstances of the killing has taken place. If the person is found guilty, then they will be executed. However, if the killing was not murder but manslaughter instead, then that person had to stay in the city until the death of the High Priest. This is what finally atoned for the killing which had taken place (pp.262-265).

Murder

In an online article by crime expert, Charles Montaldo (2015), he points out the difference between 1st-degree murder and 2nd-degree murder saying that the first is premeditated with malice and the second is intentional, but not preconceived. Usually, the punishment for murder here in America is either the death penalty or a life sentence in prison with or without the chance for parole. As the scope broadens worldwide, there are many countries that have abolished the death penalty altogether. According to the Charts Bin *statistics collector team (2011),* the nations which have set laws in place or made a commitment to not use the death penalty were 139. On the other hand, those "retentionist," or those who have retained the use of the death penalty was 58.3. There appears to be a moral code when it comes to murder. People all over the world agree that some form of retribution is necessary for taking the life of another. Some of the punishments that have been used from ancient times until now include beheading, burning at the stake, drowning, crucifixion, being drawn and quartered, life imprisonment, electric chair, gas chamber, lethal injection, firing squad, guillotine, hanging, stoning, and starvation (Lambert, n.d.).

Abortion

Some of the various laws that are identified by author Joe. Sprinkle (2006), which incorporated the protection of human life or justice for taking it comes from the laws of Ur-Nammu, being thought to have originated around 2100 B.C. This law stated that if a man was found guilty of murder, then his own life should be taken, this law parallels the biblical law found in Exodus 21:12 (p.42). In the case of *lex telionis,* known as the "law of retaliation", the application being "an eye for an eye, a tooth for a tooth." Exodus 21:22-25 says, "If people are fighting and hit a pregnant woman and she gives birth prematurely· but there is no serious injury, the offender must be fined whatever the woman's husband demands and the court allows. But if there is serious injury, you are to take life for life, eye for eye, tooth for tooth, hand for hand, foot for foot, burn for burn, wound for wound, and bruise for bruise" (*NIV)*. There is some dispute about the context and interpretation of this passage. When this is compared to other near eastern laws such as Hittite, Lipit-Ishtar, Hammurabi, Middle Assyrian and Sumerian laws, there is a referral in each of them to causing the miscarriage of a woman by striking her. Punishments may vary in the different cultures however, the conclusion of the author is that this "life" is the life of the mother, not the fetus. However, it seems clear that the value of human life is a high priority nonetheless (p.85).

Some of the arguments that have been in favor of protecting the unborn baby from the potential threat of abortion comes from the value that God places on the life that He has authored. The exquisite design of the human body reveals much about God's intention for life and when it begins. Embryonic development as discussed by Dr. David Menton (2006) in the video, *Fearfully and Wonderfully Made*, shows the meaning behind Psalm 139:13-16. *"For you created my inmost being you knit me together in my mother's womb. I praise you because I am fearfully and wonderfully made; your works are wonderful; I know that well. My frame was not hidden from you when I was made in the secret place when I was woven together in the depths of the earth. Your eyes saw my unformed body; all the days ordained for me were written in your book before one of them came to be."* Looking at the science of anatomy, the processes of fertilization, implantation, pregnancy, and birth all have complexities far greater than biology alone can explain. The truth of life beginning at conception is shown and tells us why abortion is truly murder of the innocent.

Another good resource on solutions related to human value and what can be done to protect the life of the mother and baby is the seminar, *The Heart of a Doula* (2012). In this presentation the matter of how to serve women during pregnancy and childbirth is relayed. "Doula" comes from the Greek word meaning servant. Typically, this is a woman who serves another in labor and delivery. They are known as advocates and supporters, who educate mothers and prepare them for this next season of life. In surveys that were conducted, it was shown that in every case where a woman had an abortion previously, when asked if she would have had an abortion if she had a doula, she reported that she would not have.

Manslaughter

There is a difference in motive between one who conceives to kill ruthlessly, with malice and the one who accidentally slays his fellow man. Part of God's provision, according to the Old Testament, are the "cities of refuge," as brought out by Dr. Sprinkle (2015), in his book *Leviticus and Numbers*. In this commentary, the idea of God detesting murder and having mercy on one who may have found himself in a terrible circumstance of accidental killing is shown. The man who has committed manslaughter must swiftly go to a city of refuge, lest he be caught by the family member who had the right to avenge the life which had been taken (pp. 418-422).

According to the passage in Deuteronomy 19:4-13, God shows the distinction of what must be done in the case of manslaughter verses intentional murder. It says, "This is the rule concerning anyone who kills a person and flees there for safety—anyone who kills a neighbor unintentionally, without malice aforethought. For instance, a man may go into the forest with his neighbor to cut wood, and as he swings his ax to fell a tree, the head may fly off and hit his neighbor and kill him. That man may flee to one of these cities and save his life. Otherwise, the avenger of blood might pursue him in a rage, overtake him if the distance is too great, and kill him even though he is not deserving of death, since he did it to his neighbor without malice aforethought. This is why I command you to set aside for yourselves three cities. If the LORD your God enlarges your territory, as he promised on oath to your ancestors, and gives you the whole land he promised them, because you carefully follow all these laws, I command you today, to love the LORD your God and to walk always in obedience to him, then you are to set aside three more cities. Do this so that innocent blood will not be shed in your land, which the LORD your God is giving you as your inheritance, and so that you will not be guilty of bloodshed.

But if out of hate someone lies in wait, assaults, and kills a neighbor, and then flees to one of these cities, the killer shall be sent for by the town elders, be brought back from the city and be handed over to the avenger of blood to die. Show no pity. You must purge from Israel the guilt of shedding innocent blood, so that it may go well with you" (*NIV*). Exodus chapter 21:12- 14 elaborates further when it says, "Anyone who strikes a person with a fatal blow is to be put to death.

However, if it is not done intentionally, but God lets it happen, they are to flee to a place I will designate. But if anyone schemes and kills someone deliberately, that person is to be taken from my altar and put to death" (*NIV*). It is clear even from just theses Scriptures that the justice of God is right and fair. He upheld the life He created and expected His people to do the same. The cities of refuge were Bezer, Ramoth, Gilead, Golan, Hebron, Kedesh and Shechem (2015, p.420).

The real questions that had to be answered in the case of manslaughter as brought in Numbers chapter 35 out were if there had been any previous negative or malicious encounters between the one being accused and the deceased? Were there any weapons used to suggested premeditation? What were the circumstances surrounding the death? The cities of refuge provided the necessary time and protection to exact the details in order to determine the guilt of the accused party. If someone was found to be guilty of manslaughter, then that person would stay in the city until the High Priest died (Sprinkle, 2015, p.420). So, when the life of the priest was over, it was as if his blood was used to pay for the life that had been taken. This is part of the significance of Jesus being called "High Priest" in the book of Hebrews.

War

The decree of battle sometimes warranted killing enemy peoples. This was implemented many times by God Himself in the Old Testament. How can this be just if murder is wrong? The answer is found in analyzing the context of such an order, author Joe Sprinkle (2006), make this point about war. According to the rules for war that God set up for Israel, which are stated in Deuteronomy 20:10-20, there are certain parameters regarding war. "When you march up to attack a city, make its people an offer of peace. If they accept and open their gates, all the people in it shall be subject to forced labor and shall work for you. If they refuse to make peace and they engage you in battle, lay siege to that city. When the LORD your God delivers it into your hand, put to the sword all the men in it. As for the women, the children, the livestock, and everything else in the city, you may take these as plunder for yourselves. And you may use the plunder the LORD your God gives you from your enemies. This is how you are to treat all the cities that are at a distance from you and do not belong to the nations nearby. When you lay siege to a city for a long time, fighting against it to capture it, do not destroy its trees by putting an ax to them, because you can eat their fruit. Do not cut them down. Are the trees people, that you should besiege them? However, you may cut down trees that you know are not fruit trees and use them to build siege works until the city at war with you falls" (*NIV*).

First, they had to offer peace before they attacked. This was different than other nations, which would besiege a city without warning. Then it was known that the soldiers must only kill the fighting men, not women, children or the animals. Any women they did take captive had to be given a time to mourn and the opportunity to choose marriage if they wanted to accept it. This was not the way other people treated those they were enslaving. Finally, they were to abstain from destruction, which was not absolutely needed, for instance allowing fruit trees to continue to grow. Canaanites were an exception to these rules. God instituted complete destruction in their case. These people were guilty of the abomination of human sacrifice as well as other detestable practices. (Pp.176-179). The example of "Just War" that God gave to His people enabled them to live rightly before Him and set them apart for His glory!

Conclusion

In today's culture we have seen a decline in the moral standard that God gave life on the one hand through an increase of homicides, suicides, abortions, and euthanasia. However, on the flip side there has also been a global response to some of the injustices that have been done to humanity. For example, the Universal Declaration of Human Rights, the International Covenant on Economic, Social and Cultural Rights, and the International Covenant on Civil and Political Rights have all been established on behalf of our widely shared values according to author Michelle Miaese (2004). She offers insight into the global community and its determination to see a better world for future generations to live in. For a Christian, there is the hope of a new heaven and a new earth as Christ comes back as the restoring King. In the meanwhile, the treasure of mankind, who is made in the image of God should be protected and defended. The sanctity of life has always been provided for by God because He is the author of life. In the cases where even murder has occurred, it is good to remember that the justice of God was fulfilled in the price that Jesus paid on the cross. The training of women to become co-laborers of Christ and women in their community is a goal that every church should attain to. For women who bear the guilt of abortion, a trained doula can be a source of great comfort and lead her to the refuge and renewal that is only found through forgiveness and healing. Trauma informed care is essential to the process of rebuilding in one's life. Trauma healing groups for those who have experienced abortion, miscarriage, and loss or infertility can be such a beautiful way to advocate for the sanctity of life.

CHAPTER 4

CULTURAL COMPETENCY

Cultural competency means being aware of your own beliefs and values and how these may be different from other cultures. It means being able to learn about and honor the different cultures of those you work with.

Cultural competence is comprised of four components:

1. **Awareness of one's own cultural worldview**
2. **Attitude towards cultural differences**
3. **Knowledge of different cultural practices and worldviews**
4. **Cross-cultural skills**

In your doula practice:

- No assumptions regarding what is "normal" or the meaning of verbal or non-verbal communication in any form. Please recognize that there is a wide variety within any culture of what is true.
- Be accepting and non-judgmental, avoid making comparisons between your own culture and that of others. This attitude is demonstrated by using good listening and learning skills.
- Be present and listen, use active listening skills, receptive body language and encouragement to gain more understanding and information. Validate reality if you are not sure, ask for clarification.
- Expect differences celebrate and affirm differences be open to expanding your awareness of new rituals and beliefs. Build bridges celebrate this opportunity to experience aspects of another culture; the best part of a bridge is that it allows each culture to reach the others.

Tips from the American Psychological Association to be more culturally aware:

1. **Think beyond race and ethnicity.** A person's culture is shaped by more than the color of their skin or the way that they dress. It's shaped by the person's life experiences and traditions, which may be seen or unseen to the naked eye.
2. **Learn by asking.** Don't be afraid to ask questions. People feel respected and appreciated when others take a genuine interest in who they are, so ask open-ended questions about their culture to learn more.
3. **Make local connections.** Find local organizations or venues that work with a cultural group you're interested in and stop by. Organizations like advocacy groups, religious institutions, colleges, and social clubs are great places to learn more and make connections.
4. **Pay attention to non-verbal behaviors.** The meaning behind body language can sometimes differ based on cultural norms. Pay attention to how your body language is being perceived by those around you.
5. **Exchange stories.** Storytelling is a great way to share experiences that go beyond culture. Initiate an open conversation by sharing a personal story or experience.

As Grateful Life Doulas, we want to create safety for our clients as birth professionals. One way we can do that is to acknowledge our own implicit bias when it comes to racism and prejudice, especially if we have experienced advantages because of institutional power (those who decide what resources are available) or privilege (a system of advantages at the expense of minorities). This means that we will advocate for those who are not receiving equity of care and build bridges to see systemic change. The atrocities that have occurred to black and brown mothers through history is a terrible reflection of God's heart towards His creation. We must never forget and do all that is in our scope of influence to remedy injustice wherever it is found.

BUMPY AND BLESSED BIRTH (ETHER AND GILBERT'S STORY)

Esther was a woman from Kenya, Africa who reached out to me at the end of September, and I was able to meet her that same day. We had a wonderful connection immediately! We both share faith and were able to pray together. We kept in contact and then met for two prenatal consultations, forming a birth plan. A few days before she went into labor, I brought Sara over to make sure it was a good fit for both.... it was. I had been Sara's doula for both of her children, and she had gone through the Grateful Life Doula Training, so I asked if she would like to be my apprentice for this birth.

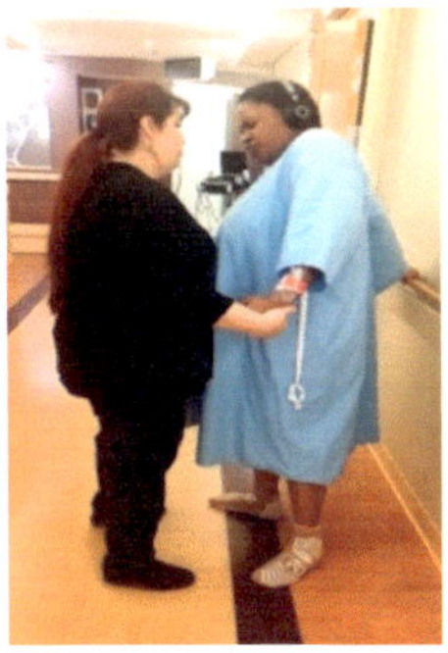

I got a text on Wednesday 12-11-19 at 4:21 pm saying some contractions were starting. She laid her girls down for bed around 7:30 pm and contractions were 15 minutes apart. I sent her birth affirmations at 9:30 pm. We texted at 1:12am 12-12-19 and contractions were about 10 mins apart. 7:41 am when they moved closer together, Esther and her husband Gilbert went to the hospital. I met them at Methodist at 10am. They did a check, and she was 3cm, 60% effaced, -3 station. The girls and Gilbert were with us for a while until labor intensified. We walked, did the stairs, used lavender oil (aroma), and when she had her next check at 12:51 pm, she was 5cm, 80%, -2. That was progress and it was at this time the hospital officially admitted her.

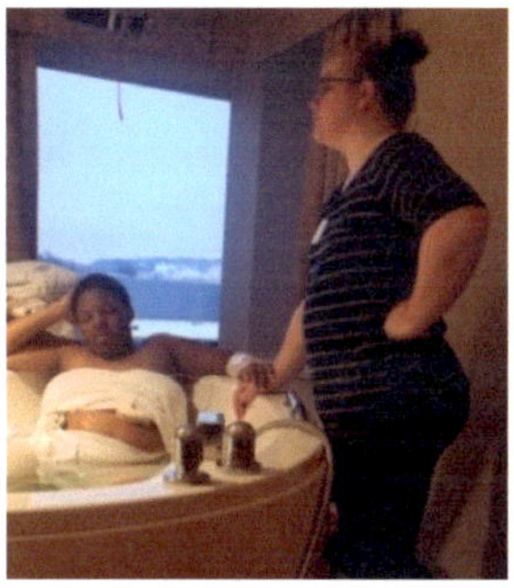

Sara attending Esther while she was in the tub.

I called Sara and had her come (2:30 pm). By this time Esther was experiencing back labor very intensely. We were "doing the dance," the double hip squeeze, and the rebozo. She was handling labor very well. Around 3:15 pm Esther got into the tub. At 5pm, they did another check- 6cm, 80%, -1. 7pm- 7cm, 80%. They decided to break her water and see if the body would progress in labor. She experienced very intense contractions, 1-2 minutes apart, so we incorporated the birth ball, oils, breathing, assurance, prayer, walking, hands and knees, counter pressure, and the double hip squeeze ... she had a lot of back labor.

At 9 pm Esther was still at a 7cm, so she went ahead and got the epidural … it was extremely difficult for her to be completely still during that time, but I was very proud of her because she went to a deep place inside of herself to gain the strength to do it! However, the epidural did not work as anticipated, and Esther was very uncomfortable during each contraction. We worked (and cried) through it for 2 more hours, then the next check revealed that her body was not dilating past 7cm and her cervix was becoming swollen. She had made peace with the idea of having a caesarean if it was needed, it was time to have this baby!

The anesthesiologist team did attempt several times to place a spinal but were unable to. So, Esther had to be put under general anesthesia for her c-section. Despite quite a bumpy ride, they were blessed to have a beautiful baby girl on Friday morning 12-13-19 weighing 8.3lbs. I went to the hospital the next day to visit and check on the family. Esther was having no problems breastfeeding and seemed to be doing very well. The girls got to hold their new little sister; it was so precious! I said a blessing over the baby and the family, praying for a speedy recovery for mom, smooth transition, peace in the home and good health for everyone.

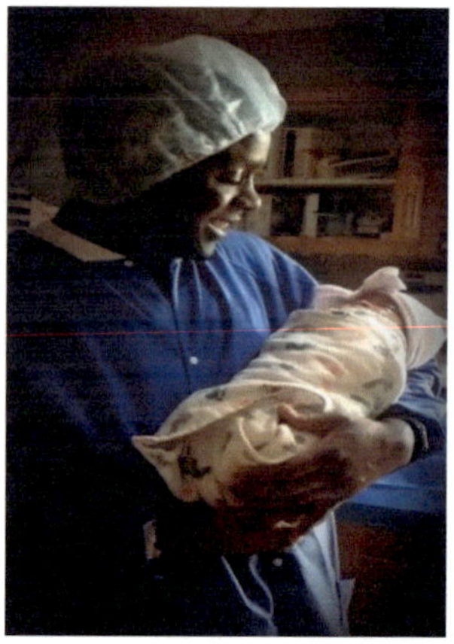

Gilbert holds his precious daughter while his wife was in recovery after the birth.

BIRTH RITUALS AROUND THE WORLD

Birth Ritual #1: Mexico

The rebozo is a traditional Mexican shawl, which is four or five feet long and made from woven material. Rebozo is a craft that has been passed down through generations and was traditionally used during birth. It can be useful during labor to help support the weight of the laboring woman. It can also be used for a technique known as 'sifting' which is thought to relax the pelvic muscles during labor, helping the birth to progress.

Birth Ritual #2: Togo

In this West African country, shouting and loud noises is believed to attract evil spirits.
So, women are encouraged to stay as silent as possible during the birth.

Birth Ritual #3: Inuit

In traditional Inuit culture, most women received support from a midwife during childbirth.
The midwives were local women who had gained experience by attending many births.
Birth is traditionally a calm and relatively peaceful affair in this culture. In fact, Inuit midwives used to whisper their directions to laboring women.

Birth Ritual #4: Comanche

Comanche women would squat over hot stones during labor. The pain was believed to provide pain relief, and these is some belief that it may also help to prepare the perineum to stretch.

Birth Ritual #5: Pakistan

The Kanash people in Pakistan believe laboring women are unclean. Because of this, mothers-to-be are expected to leave their homes a few days before the baby is due. She moves to a hut known as a Bashleni which is decorated in paintings of animals. Only menstruating women are allowed to visit and assist the woman during birth.

Birth Ritual #6: India

In Bihar, India, it is traditional for women to drink a glass of water if their labor is not progressing. Not cold, refreshing water, but a glass of water in which the mother-in-law had dipped her toe.

Birth Ritual #7: Holland

Homebirths account for around 20 percent of the births in Holland. Even if you plan to birth your baby in a hospital, it is likely that a midwife will visit your home when you go into labor to provide advice about when you need to arrive at the hospital.

Birth Ritual #8: Korea

In Korea, it is traditional for the mother-in-law to play an active role during the labor. Traditionally, the father-to-be would stay out of the room and instead congregate with other male family members awaiting news of the birth.

Birth Ritual #9: Jamaica

After a birth in Jamaica, the placenta and umbilical cord are saved. A special location is then picked out for these to be buried in the ground. Friends or relatives bring a tree with which to mark the burial spot. The young tree will be used to teach the child about the importance of responsibility. As the child grows, he is charged with taking care of the tree.

Birth Ritual #10: Ancient Egypt

In Ancient Egypt, menstrual blood was believed to be a good medicine. Following the birth of a child, the blood would be rubbed onto the baby's skin to protect him from bad spirits.

Birth Ritual # 11: Cherokee

19th century anthropologist James Mooney recorded one Cherokee ritual intended to frighten the child out of the mother's womb. A female relative of the mother would say, "Listen you little man/woman get up at once! There comes an old woman, the horrible thing is coming only a little way off. Listen, quick get your bed and run away." Cherokee women also drank an infusion of wild cherry bark to speed delivery. A woman in labor stood, knelt, or sat but she never gave birth lying down. Usually no one caught the baby who fell into the leaves placed beneath the mother, received to the earth first. Then she ceremonially plunged the infant into the river, an act that they repeated for two years. British Lieutenant Henry Timberlake an envoy to the Cherokee and the mid 18th century stated that this ritual made the children "Acquire such strength that no rickety or deformed are found among them."

Birth Ritual # 12 Black Community

Early African American midwives were important members of their community, even among enslaved individuals. After Emancipation, African American midwives, often known as "Granny Midwives," continued to work with both black and white women in rural and remote parts of the South. These birth workers traditionally occupied a prominent position in African American communities, serving as healers and spiritual leaders, and maintaining extensive social networks.

In the United States, Black women are three times more likely to die from a pregnancy-related causes than White women. These disparities are often due to variation in quality healthcare, underlying chronic conditions, structural racism, and implicit bias. Doulas provide constant communication and encouragement during labor. This focused attention can often empower expectant mothers to increase their self-efficacy and result in more satisfying experiences during labor, birth, and postpartum. According to the CDC, Doula-assisted mothers were four times less likely to have a low-birth-weight baby, two times less likely to experience a birth complication involving themselves or their baby, and significantly more likely to initiate breastfeeding.

Modern and ancient birth rituals from around the world show us just how diverse birth is.
In modern days the importance of showing respect to this diversity is imperative for new the next generation that is coming. As doulas we need to make sure we are educating ourselves on any way we may unintentionally be an inhibiting factor when it comes to our clients. For example, with microaggressions, there can be energy, behaviors, or words that we bring into the birth room that shows a level of contempt or negativity regarding a certain culture. We must instead give dignity and empowerment to every person we serve.

ALTERNATIVE BIRTH PRACTICES

1. Water birth

A water birth involves going through labor or delivery while soaking in a tub of warm water. Most childbirth centers now have birthing tubs available, though typically only for use during labor. Home water births are sometimes planned with the help of a midwife. Scientifically, water births appear to improve comfort in the early, first stage of the labor, but not beyond that. There is no known benefit of water birth to the newborn. In contrast, there may be bacteria in water that could infect a baby born in the tub.

2. Vaginal seeding

This is when a baby born by cesarean section has their nose, mouths, and skin swabbed with vaginal fluid from the birth parent. The goal is to give the baby exposure to vaginal flora (bacteria) they would have had going through the birth canal. While there may be bacteria in vaginal fluids that may be good for a baby's microbiome, it can also contain harmful microbes. For example, babies should **not** have vaginal seeding if the cesarean section was intended to avoid an infection from the birth parent (such as HIV, group B Streptococcus, or genital herpes).

3. Lotus birth

You may hear a medical term for this, "umbilical nonseverance." It's when the umbilical cord (and the placenta) is left attached to the baby, rather than being cut and removed right after birth. With a lotus birth, they are allowed to dry until the cord detaches on its own, usually within 3 to 10 days. A lotus birth is seen as "non-violent" way to transition the baby from the womb into the real world.

4. Eating the placenta

Placentophagy is the practice of eating your own placenta. The placenta delivers oxygen and nourishment to the developing baby during pregnancy. Also called "afterbirth," it's consumed raw, cooked, or dried and powdered in capsules. While it is considered a way to reduce post-partum depression, boost breast milk production or replenish nutrients, there is a risk of food poisoning from consuming placenta if it has started to spoil. Consider hiring a placenta encapsulation specialist.

5. Delay or abstain from vaccines

Some families may feel that the hepatitis B (hep B) vaccine is not needed right after birth, preferring to delay it a few weeks or months. While this may seem reasonable if the birth parent is negative for Hepatitis B, anyone with Hepatitis B may infect the baby if close enough.

6. Declining newborn erythromycin eye ointment

Erythromycin eye ointment will prevent a specific bacterium (Neisseria gonorrhea) from causing a serious infection that can lead to blindness. If the birth parent has tested negative for this bacterium during the pregnancy, it is extremely unlikely that the baby needs this ointment. However, some states have laws requiring that eye ointment be used.

7. Delayed bathing

The sooner and longer a newborn can have skin-to-skin contact with the birth parent, the better. That's why the World Health Organization now recommends delaying a newborn's first bath until 24 hours after birth in most cases. This can help keep the baby's body temperature and blood sugar in control and promote breastfeeding and bonding. However, if the birth parent has a genital rash from HSV during delivery, or has HIV, hepatitis B, or hepatitis C, it is important to bath the baby as soon as possible to remove infected fluid from their skin. There are no other known risks of infection if the bath is delayed.

8. Blessings or Baptism

Traditionally, midwives were the only women given the authority by the church to baptize infants. This was because the infant mortality rate was high, and mothers wanted to ensure the baby's entrance into heaven. Now days families may want a blessing said at the birth as a spiritual welcome or acknowledgement of gratitude to God for a safe and healthy delivery.

CHAPTER 5

PREGNANCY-A PROMISE

Fertilization	**Seed**
Conception	**Planting**
Growth	**Fruitfulness**
3 Trimesters	**The Trinity**

1. FERTILIZATION—SEED

Fertilization occurs when the sperm or seed of the man combines with the woman's egg in the fallopian tube. The instant this happens, the DNA and sex of the baby is determined. The male and female both contribute to the new life that begins to form.

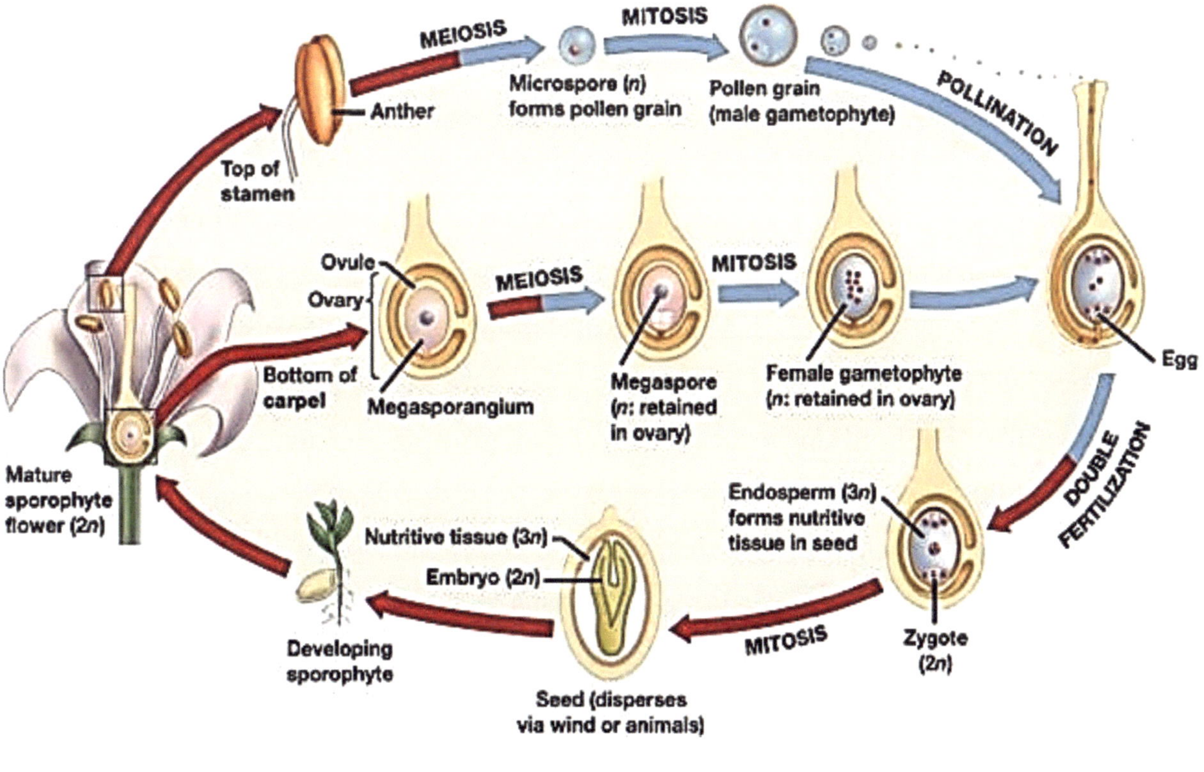

In Jeremiah 1:5 the Lord says, "Before I formed you in the womb, I knew you, and before you were born, I consecrated you; I appointed you a prophet to the nations." This is an encouragement to us, knowing that God knew us even before He formed us. Psalm 127:3 says, "Behold, children are a heritage from the LORD, the fruit of the womb a reward."

You can see the similarities between the fertilization of a plant and human beings. Amazingly we can see the unity of our Creator in how new life begins. The source of all life is in the seed. We are told in the "Parable of the Sower" found in Matthew, chapter 13, that God's Word is a seed. If it is received in faith, it has the power to produce spiritual life in us! Proverbs 18:21 tells us that "*death and life are in the power of the tongue, and those who love it will eat its fruits*." Our words are like seeds, as well.

1 Peter 1:23-25 says, "You have been born again, not of perishable seed but of imperishable, through the living and abiding word of God; for 'All flesh is like grass and all its glory like the flower of grass. The grass withers, and the flower falls, but the word of the Lord remains forever.' And this Word is the good news that was preached to you."

This is the account of the creation of the heavens and the earth:

"When the LORD God made the earth and the heavens, neither wild plants nor grains were growing on the earth. For the LORD God had not yet sent rain to water the earth, and there were no people to cultivate the soil. Instead, springs came up from the ground and watered all the land. Then the LORD God formed the man from the dust of the ground. He breathed the breath of life into the man's nostrils, and the man became a living person. Then the LORD **God planted a garden** in Eden in the east, and there he placed the man he had made. [9]The Lord God made all sorts of trees **grow** up from the ground—trees that were beautiful and that **produced delicious fruit**. In the middle of the garden, he placed the tree of life and the tree of the knowledge of good and evil … The LORD God placed the man in the Garden of Eden to tend and watch over it. [16] But the LORD God warned him, 'You may freely eat the fruit of every tree in the garden—except the tree of the knowledge of good and evil. If you eat its fruit, you are sure to die.' Then the LORD

God said, 'It is not good for the man to be alone. I will make a helper who is just right for him ...' 'At last!' the man exclaimed. 'This one is bone from my bone, and flesh from my flesh! She will be called 'woman,' because she was taken from 'man.''' This explains why a man leaves his father and mother and is joined to his wife, and the two are united into one ..." (Genesis 2:4-9, 15-18, 23-24).

Eve was the mother of all living; she was created with the capabilities to bring forth life. Our first parents Adam and Eve were tempted by the devil to eat of the fruit of the tree of the knowledge of good and evil, which brought forth sin and death. Genesis, chapter 3, tells the story: starting in verse 4, "You won't die!" the serpent replied to the woman. "God knows that your eyes will be opened as soon as you eat it, and you will be like God, knowing both good and evil." The woman was convinced. She saw that the tree was beautiful, and its fruit looked delicious, and she wanted the wisdom it would give her. So, she took some of the fruit and ate it. Then she gave some to her husband, who was with her, and he ate it, too ... Eve was deceived, but Adam disobeyed—s*in caused separation.* [15] Then the LORD God said to the serpent, I will cause hostility between you and the woman, and between your offspring and her offspring. **He will strike your head, and you will strike his heel."** This is the first mention of the messianic promise of Jesus!

He did come to destroy the works of the devil. Unfortunately, there are still consequences for sin ... [16] "Then he said to the woman, '**I will sharpen the pain of your pregnancy, and in pain you will give birth.**' [17] And to the man he said, '**The ground is cursed because of you.** All your life you will struggle to scratch a living from it.' ... [21] "And the LORD God made clothing from animal skins for Adam and his wife. [22] Then the LORD God said, 'Look, the human beings have become like us, **knowing both good and evil.** What if they reach out, take fruit from the tree of life, and eat it? Then they will live forever!' [23]*So the LORD God banished them from the Garden of Eden, and he sent Adam out to cultivate the ground from which he had been made.* [24]*After sending them out, the LORD God stationed mighty cherubim to the east of the Garden of Eden. And he placed a flaming sword that flashed back and forth to guard the way to the tree of life.* Otherwise, they may have stayed in that condition forever!"

So, we learn that God is a gardener, who creates mankind in part to care for His creation. However, before man was there, God watered the land with springs of water that came up from the ground. This is interesting because before a baby is born it is surrounded in water. Jesus called himself the "Living Water," it seems that water is a preparation for fertility and growth. Mankind was made from the dust of the ground and comes through childbirth; both were cursed because of sin.

The fruit of ground and the fruit of the womb would be affected by the fall of humanity. God being good, only created man with the knowledge of good. He never intended man to be burdened with the knowledge of evil. After sin came a need for sacrifice, God himself covered Adam and Eve with the skins of animals. This not only covered their bodies but provided atonement for their sin. Leviticus 17:11 says, "For the life of the body is in its blood. I have given you the blood on the altar to purify you, making you right with the LORD. It is the blood, given in exchange for a life, which makes purification possible." God's plan of redemption was already set-in motion, Jesus is called the *Lamb of God,* Who takes away the sin of the world in John 1:29. He crushed Satan on the cross of Calvary!

God did not want His creation to live forever in its destruction, so He made sure they did not take fruit from the tree of life at that time. Rather, He made them leave the garden and go into the rest of the earth to continue the mission He created them for. Instead, God provided a way for the fruit of the tree of life to be restored to mankind. Revelation 2:7; 22:1-2 says, "Anyone with ears to hear must listen to the Spirit and understand what he is saying to the churches. To everyone who is victorious I will give fruit from the tree of life in the paradise of God … Then the angel showed me a river with the water of life, clear as crystal, flowing from the throne of God and of the Lamb. It flowed down the center of the main street. On each side of the river grew a tree of life, bearing twelve crops of **fruit**, with a fresh crop each month. The leaves were used for medicine to heal the nations."

God is the author of life and treasures each person that is conceived. Pregnancy is a sign of the promise of new life that is growing within a mother. God had provision even in the Old Testament for restitution for any damage to a baby before it was born. Exodus 21:22-23 records, "If people are fighting and hit a pregnant woman and she gives birth prematurely but there is no serious injury, the offender must be fined whatever the woman's husband demands and the court allows. But if there is serious injury, you are to take life for life ... **if a baby in the womb is considered a life in God's sight, which means that abortion is murder of the innocent.** This does not give us the right to judge but be an extension of redemption and restoration.

Deuteronomy 27:25 says, "Cursed is anyone who accepts payment to kill an innocent person." ... Exodus 20:13 tells us "You shall not murder. [The Hebrew word also covers causing human death through carelessness or negligence]. We are to hold life and defend it whenever possible. Proverbs 31:8-9 tells us to, "Speak up for those who cannot speak for themselves; ensure justice for those being crushed. Yes, speak up for the poor and helpless, and see that they get justice." God made a promise to His people for obeying the commandments that He gave them in Deuteronomy 28:4a, "Blessed shall be the fruit of your womb and the fruit of your ground" ... The prophet Isaiah proclaims our glorious inheritance when he says, "The LORD called me before my birth, from within the womb he called me by name … I will say to the prisoners, 'Come out in freedom,' and to those in darkness, 'Come into the light.' ... Can a mother forget her nursing child? Can she feel no love for the child she has borne? But even if that were possible, I would not forget you! [16] See, I have written your name on the palms of my hands." (Isaiah 49:1, 9, 13, 15-16) ... ***our names were written on the palms of Jesus as His hands were nailed to the cross!***

God establishes a purpose for each person and prepares the way. God saved you by his grace when you believed. And you can't take credit for this; it is a gift from God. Salvation is not a reward for the good things we have done, so none of us can boast about it. For we are God's masterpiece. He has created us anew in Christ Jesus, so we can do the good things he planned for us long ago. (Ephesians 2:8-10)

2. CONCEPTION- PLANTING

After fertilization, the egg stays in the fallopian tubes for 3-4 days. Once this occurs, the fertilized egg is called a zygote, which means "yoked" or "joined together". It is the first cell of a human being comprised of the 23 male and female chromosomes that have come together. Then within 24 hours, it begins to split into many cells (mitosis) as it travels to the uterus as a blastocyst encased in the cell mass.

Progesterone is released to build up a blood and nutrient supply in the uterine wall. When the blastocyst (100-150 cells) reaches its destination then the outer wall becomes the placenta and the cells within it will be the embryo. Implantation occurs when the embryo attaches to the mother's uterus usually by the fourth week.

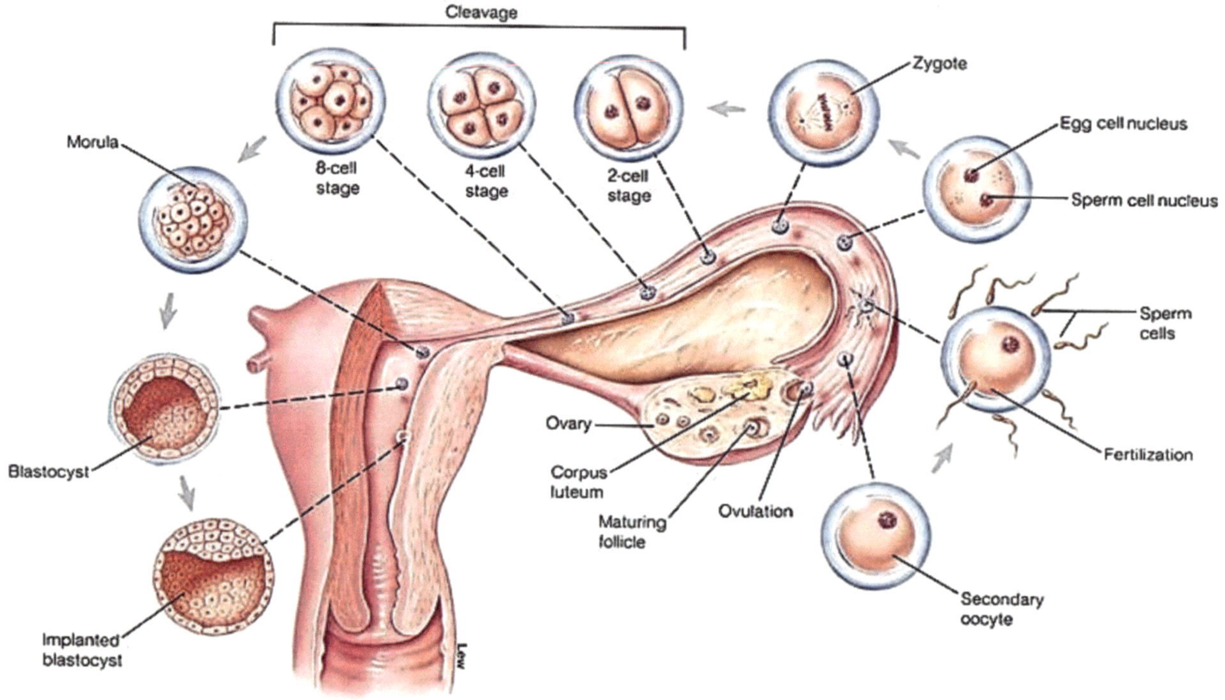

I planted the seed in your hearts, and another watered it, but it was God who made it grow. It's not important who does the planting, or who does the watering. What is important is that God makes the seed grow. The one who plants and the one who waters work together with the same purpose. And both will be rewarded for their own hard work. For we are both God's workers. And you are God's field. You are God's building. (1 Corinthians 3:6-9).

Ephesians 3:16-19 says, "… that according to the riches of his glory he may grant you to be strengthened with power through his Spirit in your inner being, so that Christ may dwell in your hearts through faith—that you, **being rooted and grounded in love**, may have the strength to comprehend with all the saints what is the breadth and length and height and depth, and to know the love of Christ that surpasses knowledge, that you may be filled with all the fullness of God." Ecclesiastes 3:11 says, "Yet God has made everything beautiful for its own time. He has planted eternity in the human heart, but even so, people cannot see the whole scope of God's work from beginning to end." This planting of eternity is within every person's soul but is hidden until its perfect time, just as a baby is hidden in pregnancy until it is born.

3. GROWTH-PRODUCING FRUIT

Just as a mother and baby begin to grow physically during pregnancy, at salvation a person's spirit becomes alive and begins to grow spiritually. Psalms 139:13-16 says, "You made all the delicate, inner parts of my body and knit me together in my mother's womb. Thank you for making me so wonderfully complex! Your workmanship is marvelous— how well I know it. You watched me as I was being formed in utter seclusion, as I was woven together in the dark of the womb. You saw me before I was born. Every day of my life was recorded in your book. Every moment was laid out before a single day had passed." Galatians 5:22-25 says that" The Holy Spirit produces this kind of fruit in our lives: **Love, joy, peace, patience, kindness, goodness, faithfulness, gentleness, and self-control.** There is no law against these things! Those who belong to Christ Jesus have nailed the passions and desires of their sinful nature to his cross and crucified them there. Since we are living by the Spirit, let us follow the Spirit's leading in every part of our lives."

Galatians 6:7-10 tells us, "Don't be misled—you cannot mock the justice of God. You will always harvest what you plant. Those who live only to satisfy their own sinful nature will harvest decay and death from that sinful nature. But those who live to please the Spirit will harvest everlasting life from the Spirit. So, let's not get tired of doing what is good. At just the right time we will reap a harvest of blessings if we don't give up. Therefore, whenever we have the opportunity, we should do good to everyone—especially to those in the family of faith."

Psalm 128:1-2 declares, "How joyful are those who honor the LORD—all who follow his ways! You will enjoy the fruit of your labor. How joyful and prosperous you will be!" The Word goes on in John 15:1-4 by saying, "I am the true grapevine, and my Father is the gardener. He cuts off every branch of mine that doesn't produce fruit, and he prunes the branches that do bear fruit so they will produce even more. You have already been pruned and purified by the message I have given you. Remain in me, and I will remain in you. For a branch cannot produce fruit if it is severed from the vine, and you cannot be fruitful unless you remain in me."

4. 3 TRIMESTERS-THE TRINITY

As a woman realizes that new life is growing inside of her, parallels can be made with the new believer sensing the Godhead moving in their life. Genesis 1:1-3 says, "In the beginning, **God** created the heavens and the earth. The earth was without form and void, and darkness was over the face of the deep. And the **Spirit** of God was hovering over the face of the waters." Just as there is a new spirit within the womb of a woman, moving in her waters; the Spirit of God was moving upon the waters of creation. And then God said, 'Let there be **Light**,' and there was light (energy)." John 1:1-5, 12-14 *reveals who this light really is …* "In the beginning was the Word (vibration), and the Word was with God, and the Word was God. He was in the beginning with God. All things were made through him, and without him was not anything made that was made. In him was life, and the life was the light of men. The light shines in the darkness, and the darkness has not overcome it … [12] But to all who did receive him, who believed in his name, he gave the right to become children of God, [13] who were born, not of blood nor of the will of the flesh nor of the will of man, but of God. [14] And the Word became flesh and dwelt among us, and we have seen his glory, glory as of the only Son from the Father, full of grace and truth." **So, we realize that Jesus is this light!** *The Word of God is revealed in the flesh, He is the author of life. The Trinity is made known right in the very beginning.*

The first trimester of pregnancy is a very exciting time! Much like the new relationship experienced in the life of a new Christian. The changes in a woman's body and emotions can range from breast enlargement, hormonal fluxes, nausea, fatigue, heartburn, feelings of stress, increased urination, food cravings, and joyfulness. From the time a person becomes receptive to the gospel, they are spiritually awakened to the truth of God. As the seed of the Word grows, it makes an impact on the person even though outwardly it may seem like nothing is happening. As the pregnancy goes on, growth continues at a rapid pace. Evidence of new life becomes apparent. The mother often experiences relief from nausea and has more energy in the second trimester, 13-26 weeks. This is a season of much change; the baby develops an awareness inside the womb. The first movements can be felt by the mother usually by the 5th month. The body and limbs are becoming more proportionate, and one can now tell the gender of the baby.

Spiritual growth also commences as someone grows in their knowledge of God, adding to their faith. 2 Peter 1:5-8 says, "For this very reason, make every effort to supplement your faith with virtue, and virtue with knowledge, and knowledge with self-control, and self-control with steadfastness, and steadfastness with godliness, with brotherly affection, and brotherly affection with love. For if these qualities are yours and are increasing, they keep you from being ineffective or unfruitful in the knowledge of our Lord Jesus Christ."

The final trimester of pregnancy lasts from 27-40 weeks. Incredible things are happening in preparation for the delivery of the baby. The abdomen continually expands making more room for the baby and giving mom stretch marks. Weight gain is normal because of the added fat the baby needs. Back pain becomes more frequent and so does urination. Typically, the position of the baby is head down at birth, however, sometimes a baby is in a breech or transverse position. The eyelids separate and the baby can see light and dark now. Relaxing begins to increase, softening the joints in the pelvis and hips. Mom experiences Braxton-Hicks and the family waits in anticipation for the new arrival.

It takes all three trimesters to bring a pregnancy to completion. Only then will the baby be ready to live independently of the mother's body. We need God in His fullness, all three persons of the Trinity to experience the deliverance from sin and a new spiritual life! 1 John 5:6-8 says, "This is he who came by water and blood—Jesus Christ; not by the water only but by the water and the blood. And the Spirit is the one who testifies, because the Spirit is the truth. For there are three that testify: The **Spirit** and the **water** and the **blood**; and these three agree." *Just as blood and water flow at the birth of a baby, so Jesus was pierced in his side with a spear by one of the soldiers, and at once there came out blood and water,* (John 19:34). *This was the birth of the Church!*

CHAPTER 6

SPIRITUAL ANATOMY: MANY PARTS OF ONE BODY

Ephesians, chapter 4, talks about how we are a part of His body and each other. "There is
one body and one Spirit—just as you were called to the one hope that belongs to your call—
[5] one Lord, one faith, one baptism, [6] one God and Father of all, who is over all and through all
and in all. [7] But grace was given to each one of us according to the measure of Christ's gift …
[11] And he gave the apostles, the prophets, the evangelists, the shepherds and teachers,[12] to equip
the saints for the work of ministry, for building up the body of Christ … speaking the truth in
love, we are to grow up in every way into him who is the head, into Christ, [16] from whom the
whole body, joined and held together by every joint with which it is equipped, when each part is
working properly, makes the body grow so that it builds itself up in love …"

1 Corinthians 12:12-31 makes it clear by saying, "For just as the body is one and has many members, and all the members of the body, though many, are one body, so it is with Christ. For in one Spirit, we were all baptized into one body— … If the foot should say, 'Because I am not a hand, I do not belong to the body,' that would not make it any less a part of the body. And if the ear should say, 'Because I am not an eye, I do not belong to the body,' that would not make it any less a part of the body. If the whole body were an eye, where would be the sense of hearing? If the whole body were an ear, where would be the sense of smell?"

"But as it is, God arranged the members in the body, each one of them, as he chose. If all were a single member, where would the body be? As it is, there are many parts, yet one body. The eye cannot say to the hand, "I have no need of you," nor again the head to the feet, "I have no need of you." … But God has so composed the body, giving greater honor to the part that lacked it, that there may be no division in the body, but that the members may have the same care for one another. If one member suffers, all suffer together; if one member is honored, all rejoice together. Now you are the body of Christ and individually members of it …"

Romans 12:4-18 also says, "For as in one body we have many members, the members do not all have the same function, [5] so we, though many, are one body in Christ, and individually members one of another. [6] Having gifts that differ according to the grace given to us to use in proportion to our faith ... [9] Let love be genuine. Hate what is evil; hold fast to what is good. [10] Love one another with brotherly affection. Outdo one another in showing honor. [11] Do not be slothful in zeal, be fervent in spirit, and serve the Lord. [12] Rejoice in hope, be patient in tribulation, be constant in prayer. [13] Contribute to the needs of the saints and seek to show hospitality. [14] Bless those who persecute you; bless and curse them [repay no one for evil][15] Rejoice with those who rejoice, weep with those who weep. [16] Live in harmony with one another. Do not be haughty but associate with the lowly. Never be wise in your own sight … [18] If possible, so far as it depends on you, live peaceably with all."

GIFTS THAT DEMONSTRATE GOD'S LOVE

- HELPING – The ability to support others so they can be more effective. *I Corinthians 12:28, Mark 15:40-41, Romans 16:1-2*
- SERVICE – The ability to find a need and meet it. *Romans 12:7, Acts 6:1-7*
- HOSPITALITY – Having the attitude of inviting others into an open house with a warm welcome. *Romans 12:9-13, Romans 16:23, Hebrews 13:1-2, I Peter 4:9*
- PASTOR/SHEPHERD – To assume personal responsibility for the spiritual welfare of a group of believers. *Ephesians 4:11-14, John 10:1-18, I Timothy 3:1-7, I Peter 5:1-3*
- GIVING – Contribute extra material resources to the work of the Lord. *Romans 12:8, Mark 12:41-44, II Corinthians 8:1-7, II Corinthians 9:2-8*
- MERCY – The ability to feel genuine empathy and compassion for individuals who are hurting, and to translate their compassion into cheerfully-done deeds which reflect Christ's love. *Romans 12:8, Matthew 9:35, 36, Mark 9:41, I Thessalonians 5:14*

GIFTS THAT EDUCATE GOD'S PEOPLE

- DISCERNMENT – To know whether certain behavior claimed to be of God is divine, human or demonic. The purpose of this gift is to prevent confusion and false teaching from infiltrating the church. *I Corinthians 12:10, Matthew 16:21-23, Acts 5:1-11, Acts 16:16-18, I John 4:1-6*

- WISDOM – To apply spiritual truth to a specific issue in a relevant way, and to make proper choices in difficult situations. *I Corinthians 12:8, James 1:5*
- KNOWLEDGE – Discover, accumulate, analyze and clarify information that is pertinent to the growth and wellbeing of the body. *Acts 5:1-11, I Corinthians 12:8, II Corinthians 11:6, Colossians 2:2-3*
- ENCOURAGEMENT – Offering words of encouragement, comfort, and motivation to help others complete their tasks and be all that God wants them to be. To speak the truth in love. *Romans 12:8, Acts 4:32-37, Acts 14:22, I Timothy 4:13, Hebrews 10:24-25*
- TEACHING – The ability to employ a logical, systematic approach to biblical study and to communicate information relevant to the health and ministry of the body. *Romans 12:7, Acts 18:24-28, Acts 20:20-21, I Corinthians 12:28, Ephesians 4:11-14*

GIFTS THAT COMMUNICATE GOD'S WORD

- PREACHING/PROPHECY – To proclaim the Word of God, which brings conviction to the hearers, so they recognize that it is truly the Word of God and respond to it. *Romans 12:6, Acts 2:37-40, I Corinthians 14*
- EVANGELISM – Sharing the gospel with unbelievers in such a way that men and women become Jesus' disciples and responsible members of the body of Christ. *Ephesians 4:11-14, Acts 8:5-6, Acts 8:26-40, Acts 14:21, Acts 21:8, II Timothy 4:5*
- APOSTLESHIP – General leadership over a number of churches, with an authority in spiritual matters, which is spontaneously recognized and appreciated by those churches. *I Corinthians 12:28, Ephesians 4:11-14, Acts 14:1-2, Galatians 2:7-10, Ephesians 3:1-9*
- MISSIONARY – Minister in a second culture. *Acts 8:4, Acts 12:23, Acts 22:21, Romans 10:15, I Corinthians 9:19-23*
- FAITH – To discern with extraordinary confidence the will and purposes of God for His work. *Acts 11:22-24, Romans 4:18-21, I Corinthians 12:9, Hebrews 11*

GIFTS RELATED TO PRAYER

- PRAYER/INTERCESSION – To pray for extended periods of time and see frequent answers to prayer. *Colossians 4:2-4, 12-13, I Timothy 2:1-2*
- MIRACLES – Perform powerful, supernatural acts according to God's power. *I Corinthians 12:10, 28, Acts 9:36-42, Acts 19:11-20, Acts 20:7-12, Romans 15:18, 19*

- HEALING – The ability to heal people in Jesus' name. *I Corinthians 12:9, 28, Acts 3:1-10, Acts 5:12-16, Acts 9:32-35, Acts 28:7-10*
- PRAYING WITH MY SPIRIT/TONGUES – To pray in a language understood only by God or by one who is given the gift of interpretation at that time. *I Corinthians 12-14 (see Acts 2, 10-11, 19)*

OTHER GIFTS

- CRAFTSMANSHIP/CREATIVE COMMUNICATION - To use one's hands, thoughts and mind to further the kingdom of God through artistic, creative means. *Exodus 30:22-25, Exodus 31:3-11, II Chronicles 24:9-13, Acts 18:2-3*
- MUSIC – Sing or to play a musical instrument to praise the Lord and to help others worship him. *Deuteronomy 31:22, I Samuel 16:16, I Chronicles 16:41-42, II Chronicles 5:12-12, II Chronicles 34:12, Psalm 150*
- LEADERSHIP – The ability to influence others in such a way that they voluntarily and harmoniously work together to accomplish God's purposes for God's glory. *Romans 12:8, I Timothy 3, 5:17, Hebrews 13:17*
- ADMINISTRATING/GOVERNING – To formulate strategies, achieve goals and guide the church in the right direction for God's glory. *1Corinthians 12:28, Acts*

Sharing our spiritual gifts helps us to be in perfect unity just as each part of the body is designed for its own purpose. Every delivery is unique because every person is special. Sharing birth stories help to pass on the knowledge and wisdom of experience to future mothers and provides inspiration to those who support childbirth. It also can be very healing for those who may have had a traumatic delivery. The aspect for the doula to keep in mind is that it is important to relay any birth experiences with the utmost confidentiality. It is a sacred trust between mothers and doulas, a special bond that is to be treasured. When mothers share their stories, then the opportunity for true mentorship takes place. Women have always attended childbirth and supported each other in the miracle of new life. As doulas, we encourage women in who they are and who they are meant to be!

PEACE IN THE STALL (KELCIE AND JOSH'S STORY)

Kelcie called me at about 4:30 pm on March 19th to let me know she thought her water had broken. I met her and her husband at the house and followed them to the hospital. Upon arrival at the hospital, she was having contractions 7-8 minutes apart. It was confirmed that her water had in fact broken and she was in labor. Kelcie utilized the bathtub to relax until her contractions became more intense and we used a birth ball in her room instead, with aroma oil. Her labor was longer than her previous two deliveries, so she did get to a point of having to lay in bed and rest in between contractions. As a result, her progression slowed down enough to have a suggestion made about a possible C-Section. She remained at 4cm for a total of 6hrs. Then a nurse had Kelcie push a couple of times, and this worked, at 3 am she had progressed into transition.

No medications were used, and at 5:05 am Kelcie told me the baby was coming. With the next contraction, the nurse delivered a baby boy. My role at this birth was to be a support for Kelcie and Josh and to provide encouragement for fulfilling their goals of a non-medicated, natural, calm birth. I was able to provide many suggestions including using the bathtub, walking, being on the birth ball, verbally comforting Kelcie, and reassuring Josh that it was fine to take a break and eat when he needed to. I also share the same faith, so in addition I read scripture and prayed as well. This was a huge benefit later in labor because when the suggestion of having a C-section was made, Kelcie and Josh felt afraid initially and so we were able to focus and pray together, which brought comfort to both of them.

When Kelcie's water broke and she called me, she was excited because this was the first experience in which her water broke on its own. She felt confident she was in labor and was ready to go to the hospital. When we arrived, she talked through her contractions for quite a while until they intensified. She was adamant about not wanting any pain medications as this was her third delivery and she had a negative reaction to the drug Nubian and was very fearful of getting an epidural. She labored beautifully, she would breathe with me during the contraction and had to be reminded to look at my eyes to stay focused. When she thought there was a possibility of getting a C-section, she was very upset and began to cry.

She was very grateful for the reassurance and encouragement that I gave when her labor did not progress the same as it had before. She had virtually no pushing with the delivery of her son, but she was in tune with her body and knew he was coming. He was put on her and then cleaned off, weighed, and returned so he could nurse right away. Kelcie did have some bleeding and pain during recovery, but she was very glad to have only Josh and me with her through her birth. Josh was very relieved that I was there so he could have a break now and then during Kelcie's labor. The baby had no trouble nursing right away.

I learned that every birth is different, and by just being there, I can make a difference. Kelcie really had her focus and I supported her in her decisions. I learned that you could encourage the descent of the baby down the birth canal by having the mom give a couple of good pushes. I put into practice some new techniques with hand movements during contractions, for instance instead of clenching her fist I had her spread out her hands and fingers each time pattered with breathing. That worked great! I realized how important it is to reserve energy when going into labor in the evening versus the daytime. Even when births don't go as planned, being positive and staying confident of each mother's ability to do what she needs to do for her birth to be a success is key no matter the outcome.

I was delighted to join this family again for their last birth too. The whole Fix family is a dear extension of my own and Kelcie is a true sister. She has been a faithful friend and prayer warrior…we have been through spiritual battle together and have seen the victory of the Lord! Kelcie has been a part of the Grateful Life team, serving in various roles and is a woman of strength who lives her love out loud!

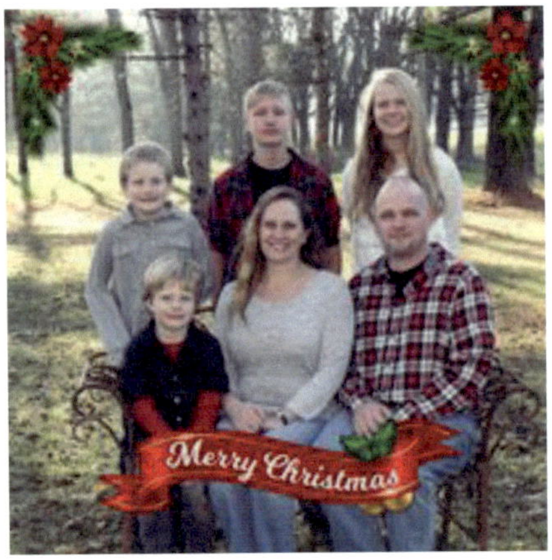

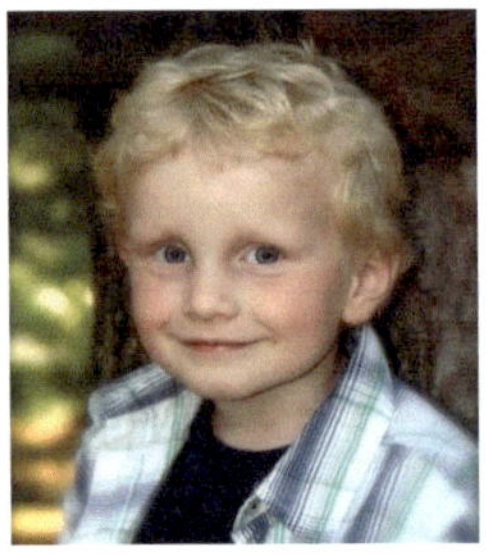

Jonathan

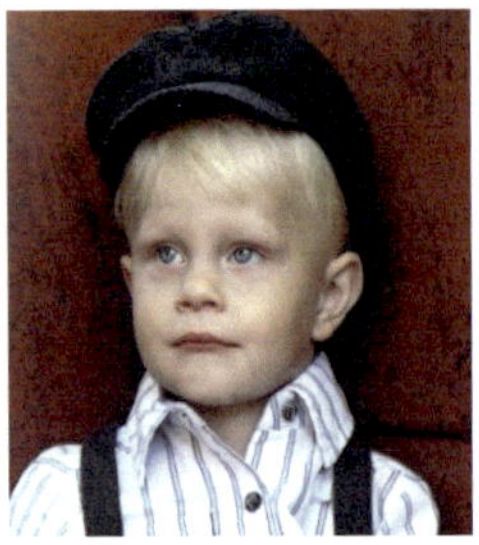

Rylin

BACK LABOR (LYDIA AND TUCKER'S STORY)

On 6-18-21 at 1:03 am, Lydia called to say that her water had broken. She was able to rest through the contractions, so we continued to stay in touch throughout the early morning. At 3:39 am we checked in with each other and again at 5:29 am when Lydia took a shower and she and Tucker were going to head over to OMC. They were admitted to the hospital at 6:51 am and I got there at 8:30 am. She was doing so well … by 9 am there were more contractions. At 9:30 am she was moving around on the birth ball. At 10:00 am contractions seem to be getting more frequent and intense. By 10:30 am we were using tea tree oil and eucalyptus and the rebozo for pain relief. At that time, she had toast with peanut butter for some energy.

Tucker is a great support to Lydia; they have a great connection! She started to have some shaking now and I am about to do some counterpressure. At 11:30 am we're all thinking about lunch. Things are starting to pick up in labor and there are some tears. At 12:00 pm the midwife came in and she doesn't feel like she needs to do anything to activate labor, the atmosphere is very positive. We did start talking about getting into the tub soon. By 1:00 pm everyone's finishing lunch and there's a lot of back pain now.

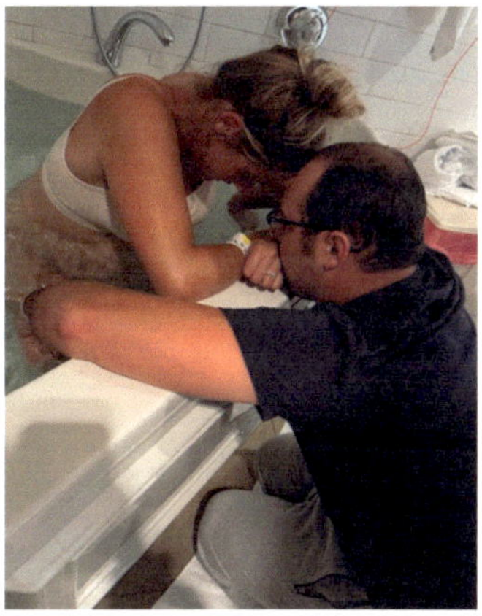

By 2:00 pm Lydia got into the tub and the contractions were getting closer and stronger; the oil is working really well! By 3:00 pm Lydia's really wants to hold her breath during her contractions but she's doing great in the tub. Tucker has been very supportive during her labor, showing lots of affection and care for her. At 5:00 pm she had a vaginal check, and she was 7 centimeters dilated and her cervix is 90% effaced. At 5:30 pm she had some fentanyl in the IV because nothing was working for the back pain.

Lydia is so brave we tried hands and knees, on all fours with the rebozo to get the baby in another position. 5:45 pm it's still very uncomfortable during contractions but she seems more relaxed. 6:00 pm she's decided to get the epidural and by 6:40 pm she was much better feeling more comfortable.

At 7:00 pm dinner was ordered, and a nurse came in to check blood pressure because the baby's heart rate had a few dips, but everything is fine. At 7:30 pm they put a catheter in her and at 8:10 pm Pitocin started. She had another check at 8:35 pm and Lydia was 9 centimeters, 90% effaced, and still pretty high at + 1 station. 9:30 pm Everyone has been resting for a while now… they checked her again at 10:30 pm and she is complete- 10cm, pushing is started!

Lydia is doing amazing she seems to be feeling enough to push effectively. We tried several positions, and everything went nice and slow. 12:03 am June 19, 2021, baby boy is born! The APGAR score is 8 (1 min.) and 9 (5 min.), she has second-degree lacerations, and repair work was done. The placenta was intact and delivered with a few pushes. The first breastfeeding was at 12:53 am and the baby weighs 6 pounds 15 ounces and is 19 3/4 inches long. I left the hospital at 1:30 am—what a beautiful birth!

1 in 4 women experience back labor. The most common cause is that the baby is in the "posterior" position in the womb, which means the head is down but facing forward with the back of the head (the occiput) pressing against the sacrum. The term "back labor" can mean having back pain felt during the contraction, in between contractions, or lower back pain that is felt at some point during labor but not the entire time. This can be very unexpected as most mothers think of the waves of contractions being felt in the front of the abdomen.

Here are some positions and comfort measures that can bring relief during back labor:

- Pelvic Rocking or Rebozo (Hands & Knees)
- Open knee-chest position (Bottoms up)
- Walking, dancing, or stair climbing
- Counterpressure or Double hip squeeze
- Hydrotherapy (Shower or Bath)
- Birth Ball

PHYSICAL—CHILDBIRTH GRAPHICS

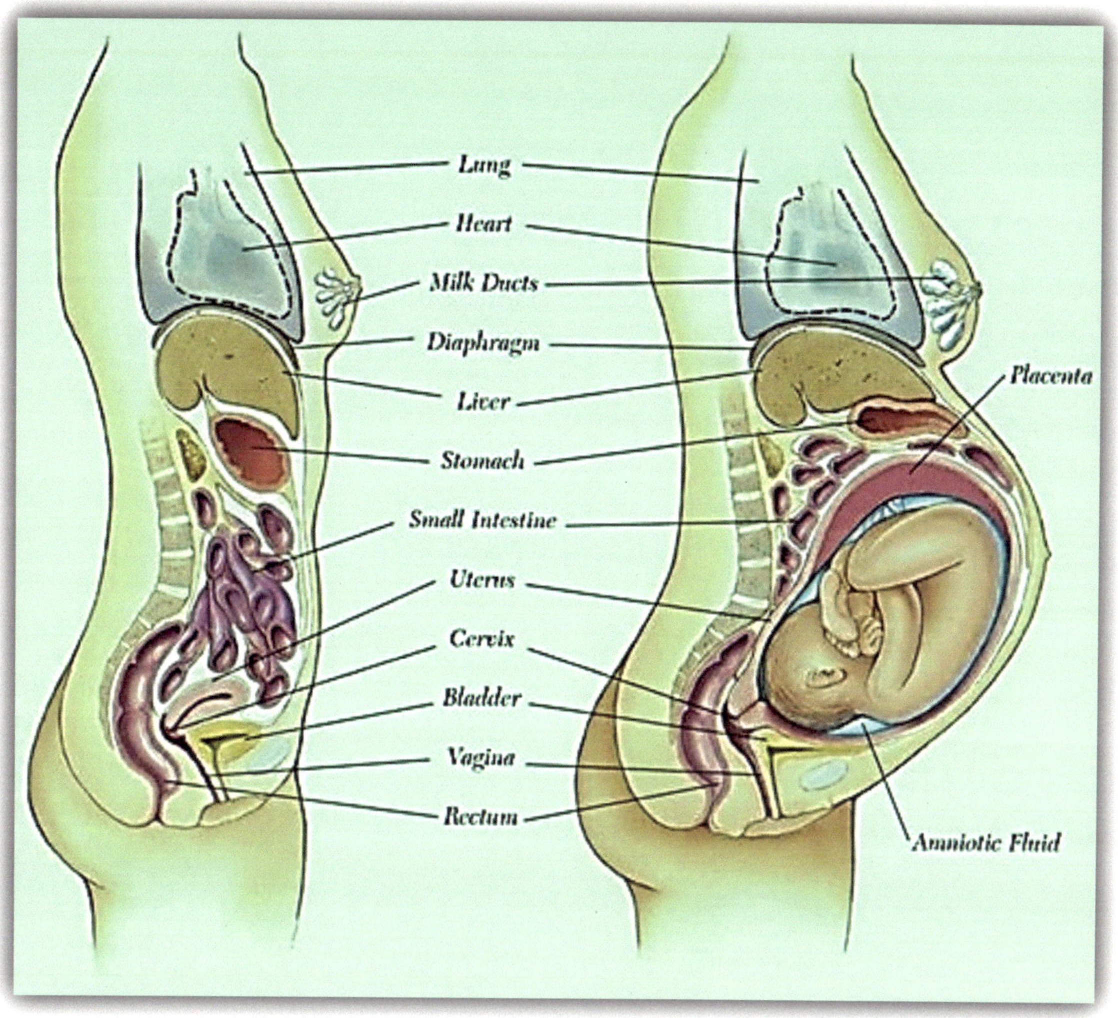

Uterus (womb) - where the baby grows during the pregnancy.

Cervix- baby will go through this opening and out of the vagina (birth canal) at delivery.

Placenta- transfers of oxygen, nutrients, and wastes take place between mother and baby.

CHAPTER 7

PROCESS-BRINGING FORTH NEW LIFE

PHYSICAL DELIVERY-3 STAGES OF LABOR

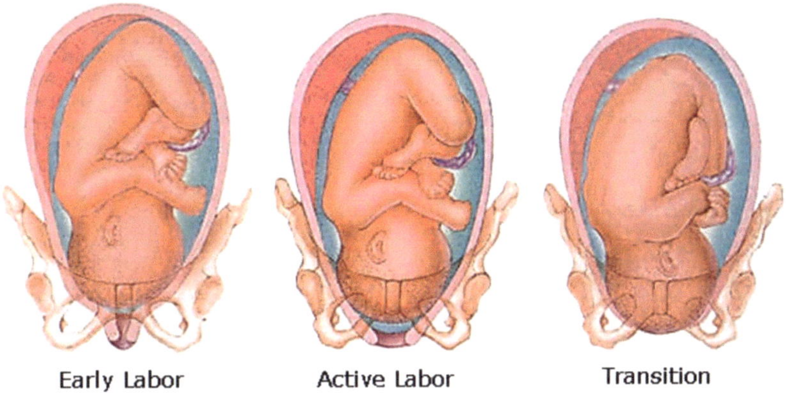

Often there can be signs of early labor. Some of these signs may include losing the mucus plug to the cervix, engagement (when the baby drops), backache, nasal congestion, Braxton-hicks, or a women's waters break. The first stage of labor begins with the uterus regularly contracting and ends with the cervix becoming complete or dilating to 10 cm. Typically, this stage is divided into a latent phase and an active phase, which includes transition. The latent phase begins with mild, irregular uterine contractions that soften and shorten the cervix. Contractions become progressively more patterned and stronger. The active phase usually begins when the cervix is dilated about 3-4 cm and is characterized by rapid progress in labor and the descent of the baby. Transition usually occurs at about 7 cm. This phase of active labor can be very intense, and it can help to have a support person, especially during this time.

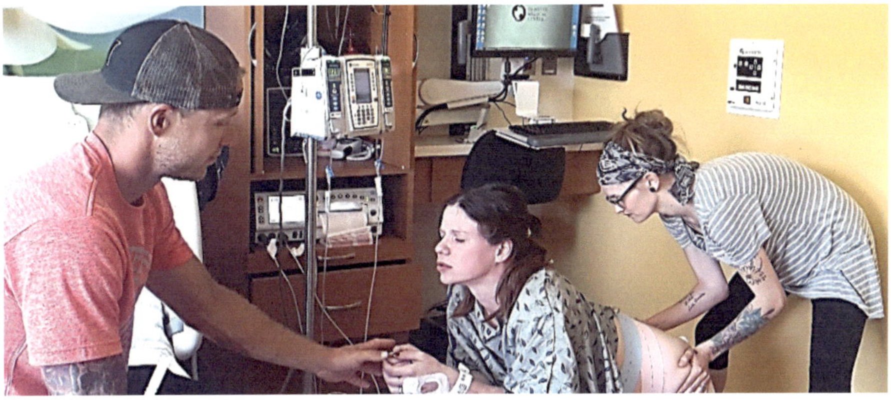

Lacy (the mother) is being supported while having back labor by her doula Eden and the baby's father, Casey. She had a scheduled induction and loved using the rebozo, double hip squeeze and oils.

The second stage of labor is the birth itself, the delivery of the baby. It begins when a woman is complete (10 cm or 4 inches). Then pushing with each contraction brings baby down the birth canal. Pushing can last between 1 to 3 hours. Sometimes the use of an epidural may inhibit this time frame time because the mother cannot feel the urge to push. Other interventions may be used when a woman becomes too exhausted to push, such as a vacuum or forceps. Some other terms to be familiar with are effacement and station. Effacement is the process of the cervix thinning out so that the baby can be delivered. It is talked about in terms of percentages, so effacement goes from 0% to 100%. The station is where the baby is positioned in relation to the mother's pelvis. It is measured from -3 to +4. A baby at -3 station is still very high in the pelvis and not close to delivery. If the baby's head is at +4 station it is essentially delivered.

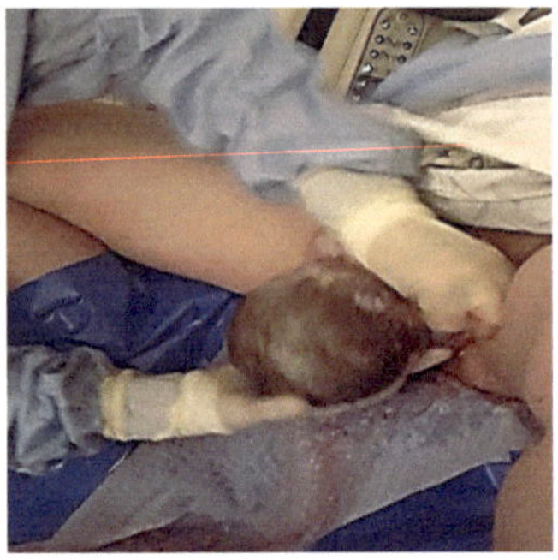

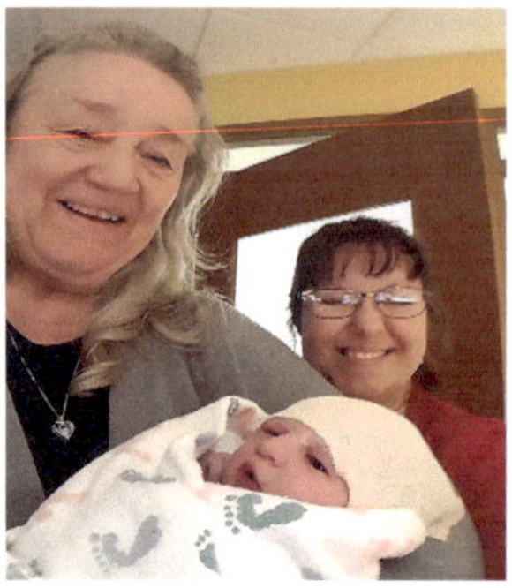

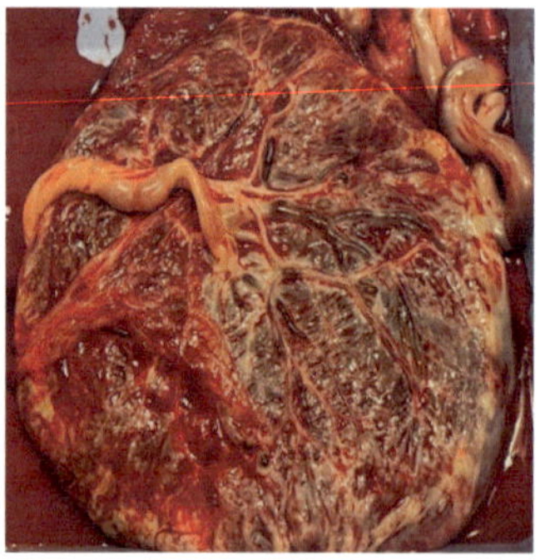

The third stage of labor is the delivery of the placenta. Usually, within about 30 minutes of the birth of a baby, the placenta detaches from the uterus and is expelled. Sometimes parents choose delayed cord clamping in order for the rest of the iron-rich blood to pass through the placenta to the baby. The benefits include higher hemoglobin and increased blood volume to fill the lungs. In the meanwhile, there is an Apgar score to assess: Activity, Pulse, Grimace, Appearance, and Respiration of the baby. This is done at 1 and 5 minutes after birth. A score of 7-10 is good, 4-6 is moderate and 0-3 is poor. Immediately after birth baby can be placed directly skin-to-skin on the mother's chest. Breastfeeding is a natural inclination for the baby at this time. This is a very special bonding time and can help with the delivery of the placenta. The journey of parenthood has now begun a brand-new chapter!

WHEN BABY ARRIVES BEFORE THE MIDWIFE

- Contact the Midwife—as soon as possible even if the birth is eminent. Valuable advice and guidance can be given over the phone.
- STAY CALM—the birth process works, most births are spontaneous, uncomplicated and normal. Try to relax. Warm the room.
- Get Mom Comfortable—remove the clothing from her lower half; help her get into a squatting, semi-sitting, kneeling, side-lying, or hands and knees position. (Not on the toilet).
- Help Her Breathe—encourage her to pant or blow through contraction and to allow her uterus to push out the baby. This will slow the birth. She should not push forcefully.
- Grab Your Birth Kit and Supplies—especially chux pads, clean towels and baby blankets.
- Wash Your Hands—(if possible, but never leave the birthing woman alone).
- Prepare for the Birth—put a chux pad or clean towel under the mom.
- BREATHE—take a deep breath and steady yourself.
- Baby's Head—the head should emerge slowly. You may see it appear at the vaginal
- opening during a contraction and then slip back in between contractions. This is normal.
- DO NOT PULL ON THE HEAD. Help mom to pant or blow but NOT TO PUSH. Encourage her to just "let the baby come" … in its own time … in its own way. The head should emerge slowly. The head will probably turn to the side. If the bag of water has not ruptured, break it when visible. Pinch the membrane during a contraction.
- You only need to Check the Umbilical Cord—if you see the cord holding the birth of the baby up. To check slip your fingers up by the baby's neck if you feel a cord try to hook your finger under it and slip it over the baby's head or shoulder (like a necklace). Babies usually move a lot and can be unwrapped from the cord once the body is born.
- Support the Head—When the baby's head will turn to one side on its own after the birth of the head. A bluish colored head is normal. The baby's body will usually come out with the next contraction after the head has rotated. If it doesn't come out after two contractions, reach in and hook your finger under the armpit and pull with the next contraction (this is usually done with the bottom shoulder, and you may have to use some force).

- Hold the head gently as the shoulders and body are born.
- Careful—BABIES ARE SLIPPERY! Note the time of the birth.
- Help Baby Breathe—Place baby on mom's chest, skin to skin and wipe the baby dry with some towels. If the baby does not begin to breath & move around after 30 seconds, hold the baby's head down.
- Wipe the baby's mouth with gauze or a clean towel. Tap the feet and gently rub the baby's back. Talk to the baby. If the baby does not breathe do CPR.
- To do CPR, place the baby on his/her back and use your fingers of both hands to lift the lower jaw from behind and beneath so it juts out. Place your mouth over the baby's nose and mouth making a tight seal.
- Breathe shallow puffs into the baby using only the air in your cheeks.
  DO NOT BREATHE A BIG BREATH FROM YOUR LUNGS INTO THE BABY.
  Remember the baby's lungs are tiny. Give about 20 puffs a minute.
- Keep the Baby Warm—dry the baby with a clean towel. Take off the wet towel and wrap the baby in another clean towel or blanket. Put the baby on the mother's chest/breast and sin-to-skin. Help the Baby to Nurse- this is very important because breastfeeding will help prevent maternal bleeding and will help the placenta separate. If the baby will not nurse rub the mom's nipples.
- Deliver the Placenta—The placenta will come out in about 3-20 minutes. Usually there is a gush of blood with it followed by some contractions. DO NOT PULL ON THE CORD! Put a bowl under the mom. Some gentle nipple stimulation may be applied to help the process commence.
- Allow the placenta to be born spontaneously. After the placenta is out, find the uterus by pressing into the mom's belly below her navel. Rub the uterus until it feels firm and the size of a grapefruit. Rub as often as necessary to keep the uterus firm. DO NOT CUT THE CORD. Just keep Mom, baby, and placenta together until the midwife arrives.
  Keep the baby on the mom's chest in her arms and keep them dry, warm and covered.
- Get the mom and yourself Some warm nourishing beverage—breathe; the midwife is on her way. Reassure the mom and talk to the baby. Keep the baby warm and fed.
  Rub the mom's uterus to minimize bleeding. This may be a good time to pray over the mom and baby or have some quite music playing until the midwife arrives.

CHAPTER 8

TEEN PREGNANCY

EXPECTED EFFECTS OF THE UNEXPECTED

1. **Facts**
   - 82% of teen pregnancies are unexpected. Approximately 57% of all teen pregnancies ended in birth, 29% in abortion and 14/% end in miscarriage.
   - Teen mothers make up 11% of all births in the U.S. This accounts for 20% of all unplanned pregnancies every year.
   - The United States has one of the highest teen pregnancy rates in the western industrialized world

   a. **Pregnancy**

   October 2001 By: Isabel V. Sawhill

   http://www.brookings.edu/research/papers/2001/10/childrenfamilies-sawhill

   b. **Abortion/ Miscarriage**

   Linda Lowen Women's Issues Expert

   http://womensissues.about.com/od/datingandsex/tp/Teenpregancy.htm

   c. **Adoption**

   http://www.americanadoptions.com/pregnant/adoption-questions

2. **Race**
   - The recent reductions in rates of teenage pregnancies, births, and abortions, show that there are still large and ongoing disparities in rates by race and ethnicity. These disparities reflect those found among unintended pregnancy rates among all U.S. women of reproductive age, which are several times higher among women of color.

3. **History**

Center for Disease Control released these findings:

- By age 22: only around 50% of teen mothers have received a high school diploma
- 30% have earned a General Education Development (GED)
- 90% of women who did not give birth during adolescence received a high school diploma.
- Only about 10% of teen mothers complete a 2- or 4-year college degree program.

a. Social- economic

The high social and economic costs of teen pregnancy and childbearing can have short- and long-term negative consequences for teen parents, their children, and their community. https://youth.gov/youth-topics/pregnancy-prevention/adverse-effects-teen-pregnancy

b. **Research/ Ethnicity**

(https://www.ncsl.org/research/health/teen-pregnancy-prevention.aspx)

c. Psychological/ Emotional

Eden, Elizabeth. "Understanding Psychological Changes during Pregnancy" 21 November 2006. HowStuffWorks.com. <http://health.howstuffworks.com/pregnancy-and parenting/pregnancy/issues/understanding-psychological-changes-during-pregnancy.htm> 17 March 2015.

d. Resources (https://www.womenshealth.gov/pregnancy/)

Special Supplemental Nutrition Program for Women, Infants and Children (WIC) – Pregnant women and mothers can check to see if they are eligible for WIC benefits. **The Affordable Care Act** – Pregnant women have more protections and options. Learn more from healthcare.gov.**Text4Baby** – Sign up to receive free text messages each week, timed to your due date or baby's date of birth. **National Breastfeeding Helpline** – Our trained breastfeeding peer counselors can help answer basic breastfeeding questions. Call us at 800-994-9662 (TDD 888-220-5446) today.

4. Risk Factors

In her article, *Risk Factors for Teen Pregnancy*, Amy Morin LCSW, a teens expert writes about some individual, social, and family risk factors that can lead to teen pregnancy. https://www.verywellfamily.com/teen-pregnancy-risk-factors-2611269

a. Individual Risk Factors

- Drug and alcohol use
- Lack of knowledge about sex or contraception
- Lack of goals for the future
- Low self-esteem
- Poor school performance
- Having sex at a young age
- Being the victim of sexual abuse
- Negative attitude towards using contraception
- Ambivalence about having a child

b. Social Risk Factors

- Pressure from peers to have sex
- Dating at an early age
- Dating older guys
- Friends who are sexually active
- Poor peer relationships

c. Family Risk Factors

- Poor parental supervision/ Negative family interactions
- Limited communication between parents and teen
- Single-parent families /Family history of teenage pregnancies
- Significant unresolved conflict between family members

5. Solutions

http://parentingteens.about.com/od/teenpregnancy/f/teenpregnancy5.htm
http://smhp.psych.ucla.edu/teenpreg.htm

a. Parents

- Have open communication about relationships, sexual activity, pregnancy, and parenting. Be honest about your expectations. Show transparency about your own experiences.
- Discuss your family values related to contraception. Give resources and provide education.
- Deuteronomy 6:6-7 says to commit and talk about what is right.

b. Society

- Recognize the association between child abuse/child sexual abuse and teen pregnancy and work to develop prevention and intervention programs.
- Support policies and programs which enhance responsible fathering.
- Expand job creation, skill building, career options awareness.
- Encourage broadcast and print media to take responsibility for establishing ethical standards regarding both advertising and editorial portrayals of sexual images of boys and girls, women and men, sexuality, and violence.

c. Community/Church

- Involve churches, temples and other faith organizations in prevention planning and having parenting and teen pregnancy programs.
- Encourage adults in the community to become mentors and make them aware of the importance of an adult in children's lives.
- More frank and positive discussion regarding responsibilities as an individual and a member of the community.
- Improve strategies for linking community members with community resources and services.
- Train lesion doulas in the local church and community organizations.

SPIRIT OF ADOPTION (EMA'S STORY)

Amy Jo was a long-time friend of mine and had been a missionary and a NICU nurse previously and had attended a DONA birth doula training and Heart of a Doula workshop. She and her husband had 5 children of their own and 2 children who were adopted. I was at Ema's adoption dedication when she was 4 years old and then served as one of her teachers in high school. When she discovered her pregnancy, she was in 11th grade. They say you can never choose the family you are born into, but when you get adopted, it means you are chosen. "Blessed be the God and Father of our Lord Jesus Christ, who has blessed us in Christ with every spiritual blessing in the heavenly places, even as he chose us in him before the foundation of the world, that we should be holy and blameless before him. In love, he predestined us for adoption to Himself through Jesus Christ, according to the purpose of His will" (Ephesians 1:3-5, ESV).

On June 14th, Ema's water broke at 8:00 pm. At 9:30 pm Amy Jo called to let me know there were no contractions yet. 1:17 am on June 15th contractions started and they went to the hospital. I arrived at 3:15 am and Ema seemed like she was doing good, she was 1 centimeter and there was not much action going on yet. At 4:30 am the hospital began Pitocin, by 6:00 am there were more contractions. At 8:00 am she was breathing through them, and we went on a walk. 9:15 am There was deep breathing, and we used the rebozo. At 10:00 am we were in the tub for a while, then they did a check at 11:30 am she was at 2 centimeters 70% effaced, and at -2 station. Ema got in bed and fell asleep for an hour and a half and then labor picked up, she was having a lot of difficulties but breathing great.

At 3:30 pm she was really struggling with pain and position and was getting tired. Her mother was there offering encouragement as the labor progressed. At 5:00 pm contractions were getting very intense she got into the shower for a minute but then decided to get back into bed and they decreased the Pitocin. She still had no pain medication, but by 6:00 pm she had a lot of back pain and at 5 centimeters 90% effaced -2 station.

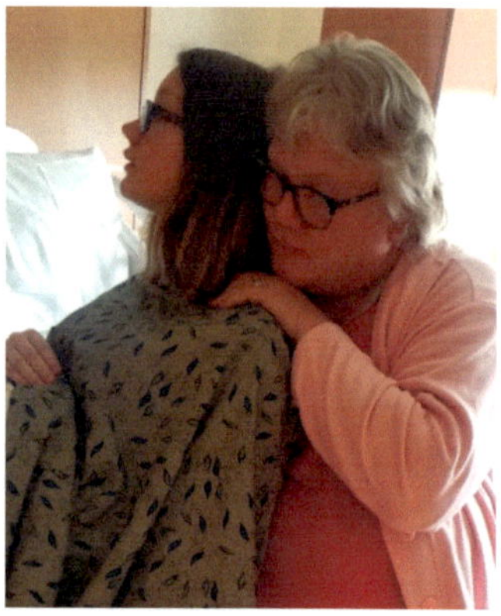

Amy Jo supporting her daughter Ema into motherhood.

During this labor Ema said some extremely funny things: "Can we cancel this one? I'm done I wanna go home, are we done now? Is the head out? Can I push yet?" I simply looked into her eyes, and I said, "Ema let's just breathe through this contraction, we'll talk about it then." At 7:30 pm, she had a lot of back labor, we did counter pressure and lots of position changes and incorporated the double hip squeeze. By this point, she was at 8 centimeters 90% effaced and 0 station. At 8:00 pm she was feeling a lot of pressure with each contraction and by 8:20 she started pushing on the floor then she moved to the bed.

Baby Oliver was born at 9:26 pm weighing 6 pounds 13 oz his APGARS were 8- 1 min., 8- 5 min. and he was 19 1/2 inches long. Ema did this birth completely unmedicated and had shoulder dystocia at the end of delivery with some repair work but was in good spirits overall. Baby Oliver was breastfeeding within the first hour. Mom and baby did amazing! After having her son, she finished her final year and graduated. Even though Ema was a teenager, she became a wonderful mother and went on to have another little boy whom I also was in attendance as her doula. Having the right support makes all the difference!

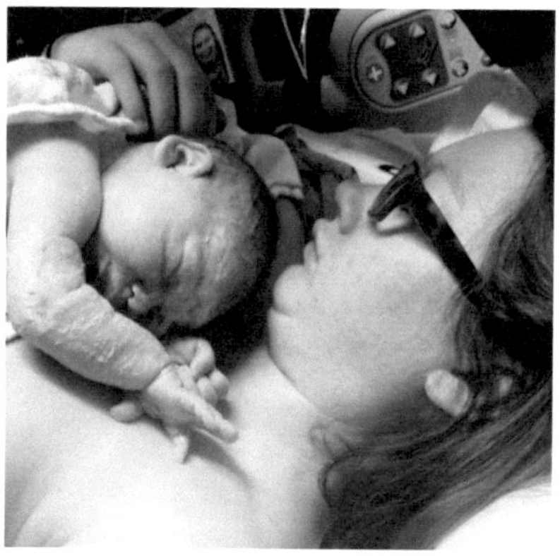

Part of what helped Ema during her labor was the parent preparation we did and doing a birth plan. Making informed choices is an important aspect of feeling a part of your birth experience. Feeling in control and empowered comes from knowing your voice will be heard, not because everything goes according to the plan. As doulas, we can equip our clients by sharing information pertaining to their options in labor and childbirth. By knowing what their preferences are, we can advocate for and support them.

CHAPTER 9

PARENT PREPARATION

Children must know that the foundation of their identity is love. They are a miracle of creation and a gift of life. They are valuable because of who they are, not because of what they do. We must see them through the eyes of truth. (Excerpt from "Making Disciples")

5 GOALS OF GODLY PARENTING

1. Self-Control: The ability to control oneself, one's emotions and desires, or the expression of them in one's behavior, especially in difficult situations. We must teach our children that they can tell themselves no, and they also have the ability to obey when we say no.

2. Responsibility: Being able to deal with something effectively or having control over something, being accountable or to blame for something, and having the ability to act independently and make decisions. We must teach our children to respect all those in authority, we honor people, not because they deserve it, but because it is godly.
The Lord places people in their position and we honor the position.

3. Humility: One does not have too high of an opinion of himself and willingly submits to authority. It is to be marked by meekness, patience, or modesty. We must teach our children, they are not the most important person. They must learn what it means to consider others before themselves.

4. Wisdom: Being wise; having knowledge of what is true or right coupled with judgment as to action; discernment, or insight. We must teach our children that in order to have wisdom, we must [honor] the Lord first, it is the beginning of wisdom (Psalms 111:10).

5. Servant's heart: A person who performs duties for others, who yields as support in action and heart. We must teach our children that we serve each other out of love and respect. The Bible teaches that Jesus came not to be served, but to serve. So, we do the same as imitators of Christ.

COMFORT MEASURES

2 Corinthians 1: 3-4 says that we will comfort those who are in any trial with the comfort we have been given by God. Our experience with God can be shared in all kinds of ways. As doulas, we can do this in very practical ways. Each one has its own special techniques which can be developed over time. Having a doula is one of the best comfort measures there is because she is able to encompass all aspects of comfort for the laboring mother. She is a co-laborer with the woman as well as with the Holy Spirit, our Helper, and Comforter.

Physical	**Mental**	**Emotional**
Birthing Ball	Aromatherapy	Relaxing Music
Patterned Breathing	Focus Point	Encouraging Words
Eating and Drinking	Information	Active Listening
Movement	Counting	Patience
Position Changes	Imagining the Baby	Kindness
Heat and Cold	Reading Scripture	Gentleness
Counter-Pressure	Responding to needs	Staying Positive
Touch and Massage (oils)	Eye Contact	Prayer
Hydrotherapy (water)	Acknowledge Pain	Quietness
Affection from Partner	Dim Lighting	Vocalization
Rebozo	Distraction	Crying (release)

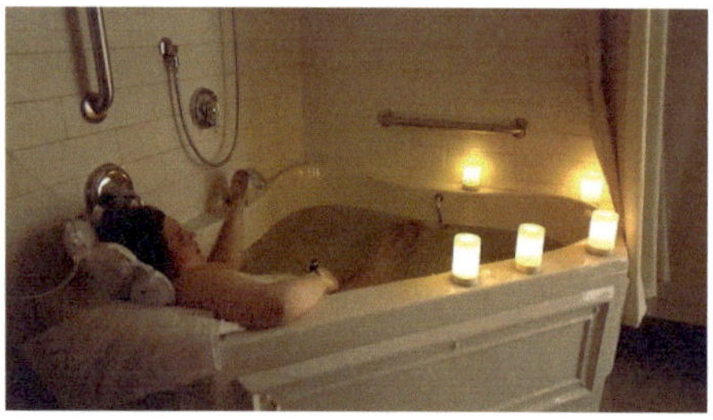

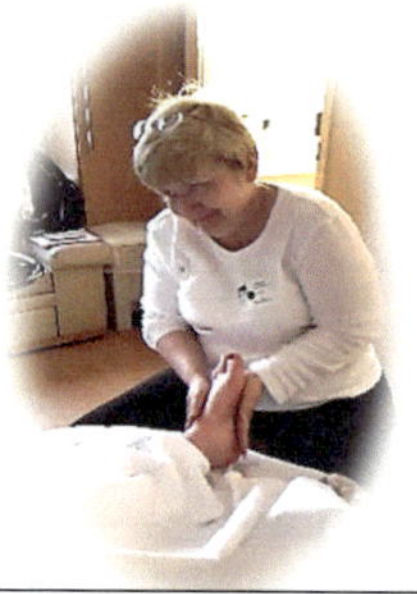

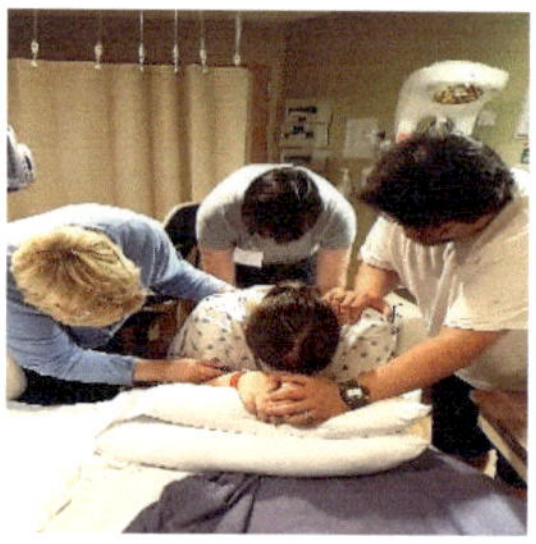

Whether comfort is found in the quietness of the tub, having a foot massage, or feeling the presence of those who care about you, it is an essential component.

BIRTH PLAN WORKSHEET

NAME:____

ATTENDANTS

I'd like the following people to be present during labor and/or birth:

Partner: ____

Friend/s: ____

Relative/s: ____

Doula/s: ____

AMENITIES

- dim the lights, bring my own music
- to walk and move around as I choose
- wear my own clothes during labor and delivery
- take pictures and/or video during labor and delivery

HOSPITAL ADMISSION & PROCEDURES

- I'd like the option of returning home if I'm not in active labor.
- Once I'm admitted, I'd like: my partner to be allowed to stay with me
- only my practitioner, nurse, and guests to be present
  (no residents, medical students, or other hospital personnel)
- to wear my contact lenses if I don't need a c-section
- to eat and to stay hydrated by drinking clear fluids instead of having an IV

OTHER INTERVENTIONS

If the baby and I are doing fine, I'd like to:

- have intermittent rather than continuous electronic fetal monitoring

LABOR PROPS

If available, I'd like to try a:

- birthing stool/ chair
- squatting bar
- birthing pool/tub

PAIN RELIEF

I'd like to try the following pain-management techniques:

- Acupressure/ massage
- bath/shower
- breathing techniques/distraction
- hot/cold therapy
- medication
- other: ____

Please don't offer me pain medication. I'll request it if I need it.

If I decide I want medicinal pain relief, I'd prefer:

- regional analgesia (an epidural and/or spinal block)
- systemic medication

PUSHING

When it's time to push, I'd like to:

- do so instinctively
- be coached on when to push and for how long
- be allowed to progress free of time limits if my baby and I are doing fine

I'd like to try the following positions for pushing (and birth):

- semi-reclining
- side-lying position
- squatting/hands and knees

VAGINAL BIRTH

During delivery, I'd like:

- to view the birth using a mirror
- to touch my baby's head as it crowns
- the room to be as quiet as possible
- to give birth without an episiotomy
- my partner to help "catch" our baby

After birth, I'd like:

- to hold my baby right away, putting off any procedures that aren't urgent
- skin to skin and be able to breastfeed as soon as possible
- not to get oxytocin (Pitocin) after I deliver the placenta unless it's necessary
- delayed cord clamping (done pulsating 1-2 mins.)
- my partner to cut the umbilical cord

C-SECTION

If I have a c-section, I'd like:

- my partner present at all times during the operation
- the screen lowered a bit so I can see my baby being delivered
- the baby to be given to my partner as soon as he's dried, if appropriate
- to breastfeed my baby in the recovery room

CORD BLOOD BANKING

I'm planning to:

- donate cord blood to a public bank
- bank cord blood privately
- neither

POSTPARTUM

After delivery, I'd like:

- all newborn procedures to take place in my presence
- my partner to always stay with the baby if I can't be there
- to stay in a private room and to have a cot provided for my partner

I'd like:

- 24-hour rooming-in with my baby
- my baby brought to me for feedings only
- to make my decision later depending on how I'm feeling

FEEDING ISSUES

I plan to:

- breastfeed exclusively
- combine breastfeeding and formula-feeding
- formula-feed exclusively

Do *not* offer my baby:

- formula
- sugar water
- a pacifier

CIRCUMCISION

If my baby's a boy:

- I want him to be circumcised at the hospital
- I'll have him circumcised later
- I don't want him circumcised

DISCHARGE

I'd like to:

- be discharged from the hospital with my baby as soon as possible
- stay at the hospital as long as possible
- wait and see how I feel before deciding about the timing of hospital discharge

Remember to talk to clients about a Newborn Care/ Postpartum Plan before the actual birth takes place, in order to minimize anxiety and for the client to feel adequately prepared.

PROVIDING VIRTUAL LABOR SUPPORT

Virtual Doula support increased dramatically since the onset of Covid-19. There are any number of potential reasons that clients or doulas may need to incorporate the use of virtual support. Here are some resources for providing virtual birth support: Zoom, Skype, Facetime, Google Hangouts or Duo, Facebook, Portal, Phone calls, Texts, FB Messenger. Prenatal preparation is the key! Have a plan A and B in case WIFI doesn't work. Practice comfort measures ahead of time. Share hand-outs, resources, suggestions about the birth bag. Clearly and specifically discuss how you will support them during various or unexpected scenarios such as unmedicated birth, medical interventions, C-section, and after birth during postpartum.

Doula Preparation- home base, quiet space, no distractions, food, chargers, no hand- held devices, and have focus on your client. Doulas Responses: Eye contact, empathy, tone of voice, unconditional acceptance, verbal affirmations, adaptability. Picture the women in labor during: Early-Active-Transition-Pushing-Birth. Is she keeping a rhythm, coping well, in distress? What help can you give? What is going through your (her) mind? How can you help the partner? Prenatal Ed., texting during the labor, verbal praise, and instruction.

- Technical Set-up — Breathing techniques
- Massage techniques — Positions, Fan
- Back pain techniques — Pushing positions
- Practice Comfort Measures — Plans if induction is needed
- Support with an Epidural — Support with a cesarean
- Contingency Planning — Electric tea lights or twinkle lights
- Massage tools — Rebozo or labor wrap
- Headset or ear buds — Comfortable chair, blanket
- Water, snacks — Affirmations
- Breastfeeding resources — Postpartum Support Plan
- Birth Bag Supply Suggestions
- When you will have a virtual or in-person postpartum visit
- When you will check in by phone or text
- Space separate from family & free of distraction
- Computer, Laptop, or tablet setup with wired internet

Feedback after a contraction … slow down breathing, good job, drink some water, follow me, ect. Limbic System and Brain Stem (mid brain — less communicative, more instinctual- match her mood. Engage her with your voice, acknowledge and validate her, don't correct her. (eg. Client: I can't do it! Doula: You are doing it…that's not validating her. Instead say, "Yes, this is so hard.") Doula care can increase the production in Oxytocin, helping the mother to feel safe, in unity, and positive.

Source: Connie Sultana, CD/BDT(DONA), ICCE, LCCE

In a virtual format, almost everything a doula offers can still be provided:

- helping to find a comfortable position
- providing reminders about rest, nourishment, and hydration
- providing guidance, relaxation, and coping skills
- helping to answer questions
- helping to formulate questions for care providers
- guiding a partner through hands-on body work that cannot be provided from afar

Prior to the birth, you may want to make voice recording files and share them. Examples are guided relaxation, meditation, and affirmations. While you certainly can direct them to apps and other sources for that, it may be helpful to start coaching them in an auditory way, creating that connection that you will be providing in advance of the birth.

Before labor:

- After choosing a format to use like Zoom or FaceTime, it's a good idea to walk your client through a session of doing it in advance of the actual Labor Day.
- If you are using Zoom, you might consider accumulating a collection of videos of positions and comfort measures that you would like partners to learn to do in advance.
- You may have to make some of these short videos yourself in advance. You may not want to wake your daughter at 2 a.m. so you can demonstrate the double hip squeeze!

- You can collect from online sources. During labor these videos can be dropped into the chat box on Zoom.
- If your client plans to give birth at a hospital, remind them to find out if the hospital's policies will allow you to provide continuous virtual support.
- When providing virtual labor support at a hospital, it is a good idea to check in advance on what the hospital's Wi-Fi connection will be.
  Hopefully their own Wi-Fi will be good enough. Oftentimes, depending on the hospital's guest Wi-Fi, service is not effective.
- Be sure that you set realistic expectations with your clients in advance of them heading to the hospital. There is always potential for Wi-Fi to be ineffective in large buildings.
- Some institutions may not have good access with particular carriers.

Birth Bag:
Be sure to share ideas for your client's birth bag. Items that you may carry in your doula bag may not be on their list of things to pack. Review items that you think they should take with them that you would normally bring yourself. For example, I usually have a fan for myself and the partner to use to cool the laboring person during the resting time between pushing contractions. The partner may not have something like that in their bag. While any piece of paper in the room could potentially be used as a fan, it is easier for you to say, "Now would be a good time to go get that fan you have in your birth bag."

Depending on regulations in your area, you may be able to join your client in person during early labor. Begin what you can of rituals, rhythm, and relaxation at home, so that your client can continue following your guidance with these at the hospital. Different doulas handle early labor support in varying ways. Many text in early labor. In the case of virtual support, consider establishing virtual contact early in labor, rather than by text. Allowing them to see and hear you early on in labor will help establish trust.

They will begin to see that you are able to provide practical and appropriate suggestions. They will hear the calm in your voice or see the calm in your face. This can be helpful in avoiding heading to the birth location too early. Because of this early labor support, they will be more likely to actually continue to access your services when active labor begins.

There are a variety of devices that birthing people can bring with them. Laptops, tablets, and smartphones are obvious options. Ideally, you want this to be a hands-free experience for them. The birthing person and their partner may want to bring a long cord for charging purposes, as well as an emergency battery pack.

Laptop or Tablet

Pros of a laptop or tablet:

- can sit on a table or bed-stand
- your face will appear bigger to them

Cons of a laptop or tablet:

- must have a large enough surface to rest on; this is often the tray table in a hospital room
- support staff often move tables to do their work, resulting in you needing to have someone put you back in place

Smartphone

Pros of a smartphone:

- can be propped on a tripod in a variety of places in the room
- can be connected to a wireless/Bluetooth speaker
- can be attached on top of an IV pole, or even taped in place with a pop socket (with permission of hospital staff)
- can rest on top of the "pump box" of an IV pole (with permission of hospital staff)
- IV poles tend not to be moved as much as tables in a hospital room

Cons of a smartphone:

- may require the purchase of a tripod
- your face will be small

Protocols for having the virtual device in the labor room:

- As new staff members join the labor team, ask the birthing person's partner to introduce you.
- Be sure that they put their device into "do not disturb mode." This will allow for an uninterrupted experience.
- Be prepared to have your device on mute, so they are not hearing background noises in your space.
- Be ready to "un-mute" it when you are providing verbal support.
- Remember that if the device you are shown on gets moved and you end up looking at the ceiling or something, they can still see you normally.
- Be aware of your resting face! Keep it calm and pleasant.
- As you speak, remember to look into the camera, not off to the side.
- Consider having lighting for your face.
- If the birthing family has two phones, you can always use the unused phone as a place to text the partner quietly.
- Remind partners not to plug into outlets with red outlet plates or unplug any devices in a hospital outlet.
- Be aware that at some hospitals, your device may have to be turned off during pushing times.

CHAPTER 10

BIRTH TRAUMA

PHYSIOLOGICAL EFFECTS OF TRAUMATIC BIRTH EXPERIENCE

The birth of a baby is supposed to be a time for celebration and excitement; however, this is not the experience that everyone has. Instead of a moment that brings the fulfillment of long-awaited anticipation, it is filled with terror, helplessness, and pain. Childbirth is a rite of passage in many cultures and brings honor, blessing and empowerment to women. So, what happens when the labor does not go as planned or perhaps there is a significant injury to the mother or baby?
The effects can be damaging physiologically when there has been a traumatic birth experience. These effects can be experienced by the mother, father, any support person or professional in attendance, and the baby.

I am a certified birth doula through DONA International and have seen the spectrum of birth experiences. The first birth I attended before certification was that of my 18-year-old sister. She had a very difficult pregnancy, being hospitalized 3 times for a week each visit because she was so sick. When it came time for her to deliver, she was in labor for 72 hours, pushed four hours altogether, had a double episiotomy, and ultimately my niece was born vaginally using forceps. Not only was the mother affected by this traumatic birth experience, but so was the father and their daughter who had just been born. The parents were not being well informed at the time things were happening in the delivery room. This caused a lot of fear and panic in the father especially because he was not sure if the safety of the mother and baby were at risk. His daughter had severe pain and cried the whole stay in the hospital. It was not until they took her in for a chiropractic adjustment that the baby felt relief. Because of the difficult time she had in the birth canal, the baby had some neck and back misalignments. My sister thought she was going to die and in her own words described the experience as "Having an out-of-body experience where you still feel everything and it's so painful, but you can't get away!" As a result, she did not properly bond with her daughter due to the many complications surrounding the birth and recovery; thus, forcing her focus to be on trying to stay alive.

Witnessing this birth trauma made an impact on me as her sister, as well. I needed to process the experience with other birth professionals years later and learned how incredibly important it is to be aware of how to prevent birth trauma when possible. This was a part of what led me to become a doula!

Post-Traumatic Stress Disorder

According to Penny Simkin PT (2015), the founder of PATTCh, between 25 and 34 percent of women say that their birth experience was traumatic. This means they felt like their life, or the life of the baby was at risk during delivery. Studies show that as many as 9 percent of women may develop Post-Traumatic Stress Disorder (PTSD) after having a traumatic birth. This is called "Birth Trauma. "In her article "Birth Trauma: Posttraumatic Stress Disorder After Childbirth" (2013), Grace Helen Zimmerman, a registered nurse and birth doula, points out the prevalence of PTSD in mothers who have recently given birth. Some of the ongoing symptoms one may have as a result of PTSD may be strong emotional reactions when thinking about the birth, nightmares, flashbacks, difficultly sleeping or concentrating, panic attacks, detachment from the baby or partner, depression and fear about the future. It can be very difficult to determine whether one has PTSD as a direct result from birth trauma or if it has another source because many other disorders have the same effects on mood, emotions, and physical symptoms. Zimmerman then discussed the causes and risk factors related to birth trauma. Sichel and Driscoll (1999) pointed out that reproductive hormone levels during the postpartum period and perceived trauma on the part of the mother leave her very open to PTSD (as cited in Zimmerman, p.62).

One may consider any of the following traumatic experiences during delivery, unexpected medical interventions, intolerable pain, uncaring attendants, an unsafe or inhumane environment, and the potential for injury or death for the mother or baby. Gamble and Creedy (2005) were apart of determining risk factors so that identifying pregnant women who were at risk would be easier. In this way providers could give more care and education to these women. If a woman had traumatic experiences or a history of depression, this increased her chances of having PTSD.

When a woman is preparing to give birth, her care providers should be identifying any factors that may impose a risk in developing PTSD. As she progresses in her pregnancy, education and resources should be made available to her. When the time comes for her to deliver her baby, careful records should be kept about how things are going. If there is any time when the mother is left feeling out control or if a traumatic event should happen, then those notes can be passed on to her caretakers. At the postpartum appointment, a screening can be done if the mother is experiencing any symptoms of PTSD (p. 64).

If a diagnosis of PTSD is founded, then cognitive and complementary treatment is needed. Cognitive behavioral therapy (CBT) gives the woman a chance to talk about her birth experience. It helps the mother better cope with stressful events and negative emotions. Deep breathing and relaxation can be helpful benefits during this time. They reduce anxiety and make it easier for the mother to release her feelings through talking about them. If one does not meet the requirements for PTSD for one reason or the other, they may be diagnosed with Post-Traumatic Stress Symptoms (PTSS) or Post-Traumatic Stress Effects (PTSE) or even Partial Post Traumatic Stress Disorder (PPTSD). Recovery is possible, with time and dedicated caregivers. Knowing helpful solutions is key. Finding those who will listen to your experience and support you will give an added strength. Also getting good sleep, having a healthy diet, massage, exercise, self-help books, websites, and counseling.

Child Sexual Abuse and Depression

Factors other than specifically PTSD regarding traumatic birth experience are child sexual abuse and depression. Simkin and Klaus (2004) noted that one in five women have been sexually abused as children. During the course of childbirth, a woman can have painful childhood memories surface. Other experiences that may trigger a negative response are vaginal examinations, having to be undressed in front of others, and feeling pelvic pain (as cited in Zimmerman, 2013, p. 62). According to author Victor Vieth in his article "What Would Walther Do? Applying Law and Gospel to Victims and Perpetrators of Child Sexual Abuse" (2012), feeling helpless is another effect of sexual abuse because once a perpetrator has shown that he has control over the body of a victim, she may let go of the tendency to exert control over the situation. Giving birth is one of the most empowering experiences a woman can have, so to be in a situation where she feels helpless is detrimental to her. This can even transfer into her mothering abilities, if she thinks she is not a capable parent because of her perceived failure in giving birth the way she planned. The Child Sexual Abuse Accommodation Syndrome (CSAAS) is a useful tool in recognizing signs of sexual abuse. Dr. Roland Summit from UCLA is credited for coming up with this model in 1983. He proposes that sexual abuse has these factors present: Secrecy, Helplessness, Entrapment and Accommodation, Delayed and Unconvincing Disclosure, Retraction (Vieth, 2012, p. 258). Factors other than specifically PTSD regarding traumatic birth experience are child sexual abuse and depression. Simkin and Klaus (2004) noted that one in five women have been sexually abused as children. During childbirth, a woman can have painful childhood memories surface.

Other experiences that may trigger a negative response are vaginal examinations, having to be undressed in front of others, and feeling pelvic pain (as cited in Zimmerman, 2013, p. 62). According to author Victor Vieth in his article "What Would Walther Do? Applying Law and Gospel to Victims and Perpetrators of Child Sexual Abuse" (2012), feeling helpless is another effect of sexual abuse because once a perpetrator has shown that he has control over the body of a victim, she may let go of the tendency to exert control over the situation. Giving birth is one of the most empowering experiences a woman can have, so to be in a situation where she feels helpless is detrimental to her. This can even transfer into her mothering abilities if she thinks she is not a capable parent because of her perceived failure in giving birth the way she planned. Child Depression was found to reduce a woman's chance to be able to deal with stressful situations. It can also change the way she sees herself or her baby, leading to the lack of connection needed in proper bonding patterns.

Attachment

In the article" Trauma, Attachment, and Spirituality: A Case Study," authors L.E. Maltby and T.W. Hall (2012) show the interaction between the factors of trauma, attachment, and spirituality (p. 302). In "Trauma, Attachment, and Spirituality: A Case Study," authors L.E. Maltby and T.W. Hall (2012) show the interaction between the factors of trauma, attachment, and spirituality (p. 302). It is unfortunate when a secure attachment is not made at birth and instead insecure ones become present. Some of these may include dissociation, impaired self-development, and disorganized attachment.

When a person goes through a point of trauma, the implicit and explicit systems become separated in order to deal with the stress one is under at that moment. Hormones called glucocorticoids are sent into the brain so that the energy needed will be there in order to cope with the trauma. The mind is created with special defense mechanisms, such as coping by separating from events that are too painful.

Fathers

Mothers are not the only ones who experience traumatic birth. Sometimes fathers are impacted negatively by watching their loved one go through so much pain. Christian Inglis (2014), a psychology researcher, found that 11.5 percent of fathers had symptoms of PTSD, and as much as 20 percent experienced depression. Feeling unprepared, helpless, and out of control during labor and delivery leads many of these men to have higher levels of stress, anxiety, and detachment from their babies. What Inglis has suggested is that the father needs to be communicated with during labor and delivery, so he feels equipped with the knowledge of what is transpiring. He also recommends that fathers should attend childbirth classes in order to have as much preparation as possible. A father may be afraid of possible outcomes during childbirth, however, if he feels like he knows what is happening and why then he can partner with the mother as the labor progresses. After the birth of the baby, it would be a good idea to continue the care of the father and make sure he is all right too.

Secondary Traumatic Stress

Sooner or later those who serve professionally as support for the laboring mother are bound to see births that do not go as planned. Doulas, (designated labor coaches) are sometimes traumatized in the midst of circumstances during childbirth that are unavoidable. In her article, "Help for Doulas Who Are Traumatized by Births They Attend" Penny Simkin, PT, CD(DONA) (2015) brings out that unexpected complications or tragedy during birth can leave the doula feeling frightened and helpless. As they witness physical injury, uncaring treatment from hospital staff or partner, the humiliation of the mother, protocol, and procedure instead of protection, shattered hopes for a perfect birth experience, and parents who are exhausted with their efforts, doulas may have a lasting emotional impact of anger, fear, feeling alone, and they may feel somewhat responsible for the birth plan not being followed. In some cases, doulas have developed “Secondary Traumatic Stress (STS). She may have symptoms that include insomnia, nightmares, guilt, reoccurring thoughts about what she could have done differently, a need to talk to someone who can clarify, anger, avoidance of the hospital, anxiety, withdrawal from friends, and considerations of quitting doula work. For these doulas, it is important to regain a clear perspective and deal with any negative psychological effects in order to go forward.

Some helpful tips for those who have witnessed traumatic births would be to process the birth experience with the parents if appropriate, talk with the doctors or nurses who may have been on staff that night, write down anything which was disturbing or did not meet expectations, a good source of support is another doula and finally if lingering feelings persist, consult a trauma therapist or attend a group which deals with trauma. These are just a few ways to rebuild oneself confidence after being affected by a traumatic birth experience. Another useful tool which to guide one’s journey through healing and knowledge about this topic is the book entitled “Traumatic Childbirth” by authors Cheryl Tatano Beck, Jeanne Watson Driscoll, and Sue Watson (2013). This is a collaboration of three different perspectives all integrated for the common goal of shedding light on the research about birth trauma and the psychological effects it brings. There is a wide range of information regarding therapeutic approaches, and the perspectives of mothers, partners, and clinicians.

Traumatized Infant

One must not forget that the baby is also being affected during a traumatic birth experience. The earlier traumas one experiences in life can leave lasting imprints as one develops and matures according to Lorri Craig (2015), a psychologist. In her article,” Can a Difficult Birth Create Psychological Problems Later?” she reveals that as a baby is birthed, he/she is going through tangible changes in where he/she is physically and how he/she is feeling. The emotional state of the mother can be transferred to the baby during birth and the impression it can leave may be significant. Being squeezed through the birth canal, possibly stuck in the same position for hours, separated from the only environment the baby has known, having the umbilical cord around the neck producing a lack of oxygen, having forceps used in delivery, and any panic or fear expressed by others, are all different ways that trauma can be experienced by the infant. Some psychological effects of having a traumatic birth experience are having a higher degree of anxiety and/or aggression, being afraid of abandonment, and anger.

Fortunately, there are some treatments available, EMDR [Eye Movement Desensitization and Reprocessing], EFT [Emotional Freedom Technique], and AIT [Advanced Integrative Therapy]. All of these can be very helpful techniques in going forward from birth trauma for those it affects.

Risk Factors

Some of the potential risk factors that increase one's probability of experiencing a traumatic birth that was found in the last decade, by researchers in the United Kingdom (Bailham and Joseph 2003) and the Netherlands (Olde et al 2006). They found that women are more likely to develop symptoms if they have premature births or miscarriages, difficult deliveries that require instrumental interventions, emergency cesarean sections, feelings of fear for the well-being of their babies or for themselves, feelings of helplessness or a lack of control during labor, a history of other traumatic experiences, such as sexual abuse, a history of psychological problems or trait anxiety, insufficient social support from partners and/or staff.

Cognitive Distortions

Sometimes distorted thoughts can leave you anxious, and depressed, and damage your relationships after delivery. These may also be a sign of Post-Partum Depression. It's important to be aware of any symptoms or thought patterns that are not normal for the mother during the postpartum period, so she can talk to her medical provider or take steps to ensure her mental health after the birth of her baby.

1. ALL-OR-NOTHING THINKING: You see things in black-and-white categories. If your performance falls short of perfect, you see yourself as a total failure.
2. OVERGENERALIZATION: A single negative event as a never-ending pattern of defeat.
3. MENTAL FILTER: You pick out a single negative detail and dwell on it exclusively so that your vision of all reality becomes hindered.
4. DISQUALIFYING THE POSITIVE: You reject positive experiences by insisting they "don't count" for some reason or another. In this way, you can maintain a negative belief.

5. JUMPING TO CONCLUSIONS: You make a negative interpretation even though there are no definite facts that convincingly support your conclusion.
    a. Mind Reading: You conclude that someone is reacting negatively to you.
    b. Fortune Telling: You anticipate that things will turn out badly.
6. MAGNIFICATION (CATASTROPHIZING) OR MINIMIZATION: Exaggerate the importance of things, or you inappropriately shrink things.
7. EMOTIONAL REASONING: You assume that your negative emotions necessarily reflect the way things really are: "I feel it, therefore it must be true."
8. SHOULD STATEMENTS: You try to motivate yourself with "Shoulds," "Shouldn't," "Must" and "Ought's." The emotional consequence is guilt. When you direct should statements toward others, you feel anger, frustration, and resentment.
9. LABELING AND MISLABELING: This is an extreme form of overgeneralization. Instead of describing your error, you attach a negative label to yourself: "I'm a loser." When someone else's behavior rubs you the wrong way, you attach a negative label to him: "He's a lazy louse." Mislabeling involves describing an event with language that can be highly colored and emotionally loaded.
10. PERSONALIZATION: You see yourself as the cause of some negative external event for which, in fact, you were not primarily responsible.

Labor Support

Research shows that women in labor benefit from a supportive companion, who is continuously present, who praises and touches the women, and who explains what is going on (Trevathan 1999). When women receive such social support, they have better childbirth experiences. They have shorter labors and fewer medical interventions (Scott et al 1999). These women also report less pain and feel they have more control over the process (Langer et al 1998). They also have better postpartum experiences. In several controlled studies (summarized in Klaus et al 1992), women admitted to maternity wards were assigned to receive either enhanced social support or routine hospital procedures only. Women who received enhanced social support had easier childbirths. Six weeks later, they also showed lower anxiety levels, lower rates of depression, higher self-esteem, increased rates of breastfeeding, more time spent with their infants, more positive feelings about their families.

Grateful Life Ministries builds up communities with trained doulas to reduce birth trauma and see families supported in their pregnancy, labor, postpartum and parenting!

We also need those who will walk alongside others on the spiritual journey of new life through deliverance and discipleship.

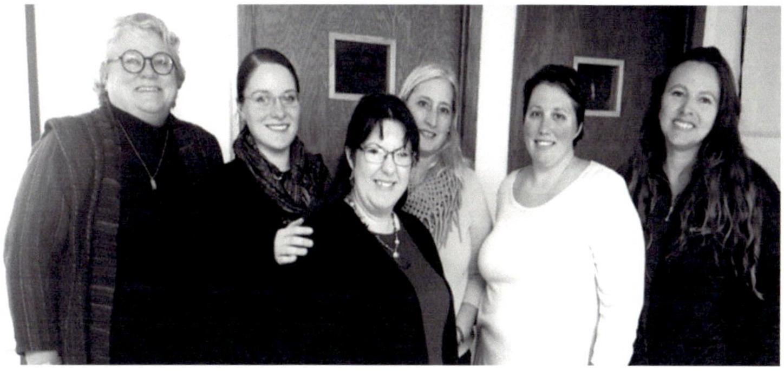

Above: Amy Jo, Abby, Jessica, Jill, Amanda, and Jen took the "Heart of a Doula" workshop by Grateful Life Ministries.

Below: Eden and Jessica co-laboring in the birth experience of a friend. They took turns providing counterpressure and doing the double hip squeeze.

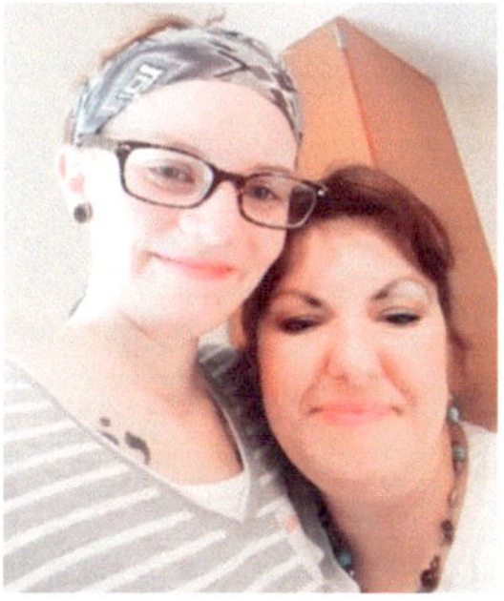

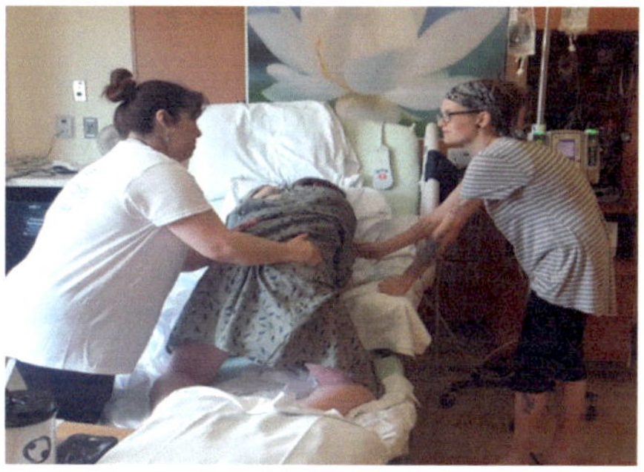

The ABC objectives for us in reducing birth trauma are:

- **Awareness** about birth trauma prevention for those more at risk, including people of color.
- **Bridge-building** skills to advance community resources related to techniques for parent support.
- **Communication** methods and tools to use for trauma healing in childbirth experiences.

We want to see families come to a place of wholeness…trauma healing groups can be a wonderful resource to any birth community. Grateful Life Ministries has partnered with the Trauma Healing Institute for training and certification as facilitators of trauma healing. There are many tools for healing along our journey and those we can connect with while on this path. For more information, please go to https://traumahealingbasics.org/

CHAPTER 11

DELIVERANCE: BEING BORN AGAIN

SPIRITUAL DELIVERANCE FOR THE BODY-SOUL-SPIRIT

We need deliverance in our Body, Soul, and Spirit. We are a three-part being:
Body, Soul, Spirit (1 Thessalonians 5:23). We are made in the image and likeness of God. God the Father is the creator; God the Holy Spirit is present to move; God the Son, Jesus, is the light; the very Word of God. God is a three-part being, just as we are. (Genesis 1: 1-3, 26, 27). God's universe has order; He created it to work that way. Man was designed with three distinct, yet integrated parts. They were made to function in proper order and relationship. Man was created to have his spirit in control of his being.

Spirit:

The eternal part of us that will continue beyond our earthly life. We are born physically,
then born again spiritually (John 3).

Soul:

"Those which breaths" or "Life"- **mind** (how we think), emotions (how we feel),
and our **will** (how we choose.)

Body:

God formed man from the dust of the ground (Genesis 1). It houses our spirit and soul during our earthly life.

Deliverance means to make a complete break from the past, to be set free. In the Bible, there are several categories where cleansing or deliverance is needed. There is also a pathway to freedom that is shown for each one:

Deliverance	Pathway	Scripture
1. Sickness	Pray in Faith	James 5:14
2. Religion	Law of Liberty	James 1:25
3. Demonic	Cast out	Mark 16:17
4. Sin	Confess	1 John 1:9
5. Trauma	Healing	Luke 4:18

During childbirth, the baby is being delivered. Our deliverance occurs when we become born again spiritually. John chapter 3:1-6 tells us about being born again. "Now there was a man of the Pharisees named Nicodemus, a ruler of the Jews. This man came to Jesus by night and said to him, 'Rabbi, we know that you are a teacher come from God, for no one can do these signs that you do unless God is with him.' Jesus answered him, 'Truly, truly, I say to you, unless one is born again, he cannot see the kingdom of God.' Nicodemus said to him 'How can a man be born when he is old? Can he enter a second time into his mother's womb and be born?' Jesus answered, 'I say to you, unless one is born of water and the Spirit, he cannot enter the kingdom of God. That which is born of the flesh is flesh, and that which is born of the Spirit is spirit.'"

It is important to understand that rebirth happens in our spirit. Our soul and body are not reborn. Being born again and the freeing of our soul are two separate matters. Remember our spirit is justified and our soul needs **sanctification**- (Transformation process). **Justification**- (being completely pure before God, like we never sinned) happens in our spirit happens at salvation but being sanctified is a process. It is important to distinguish between possession. and bondage. When we receive Christ, the Holy Spirit takes possession of our spirit. 1 Corinthians 3:16, "Don't you know you are God's temple and that God's Spirit lives inside of you." Therefore, a Christian cannot be demon-possessed. Possession means one who controls your spirit, this means God, your soul or the demonic. Bondage in contrast is what controls the soul. Therefore, bondages like addictions, anger, rejection, fear, lust, and bitterness involve our minds, will, and emotions. Although a believer is not demon-possessed, areas of bondage can and do exist.

We as believers need to know the ways demonic activity can influence our lives. Just as germs can affect our physical body, demons can affect us spiritually. The scripture shows us that when we are tempted and sin, we open the door to the devil and his demon forces.

Satan knows that he can't possess the church, so instead he looks for all the ways to influence and manipulate it. Ephesians 4:17 tells us not to give any place or foothold to the devil. The word Place in Greek is *Topias*—which means ground or territory. When we sin repeatedly in a specific area, we give the devil a place in our lives. The devil cannot be everywhere at once, so he relies on our flesh - soul not surrendered- (mind, will, emotions) and demons to work out his plans.

When we don't choose cleansing and deliverance, four things happen:

1. Distortion—Romans 7:19
2. Corruption—Romans 1:21-22
3. Blindness—Ephesians 4:18
4. Hardness—Ephesians 4:19

Temptation does not come from God, James 1:13-15 says, "When tempted no one should say God is tempting me, for God cannot be tempted by evil, nor does He tempt anyone. Each one is tempted when he is drawn away by his own desires and enticed. When desire has conceived, it gives birth to sin and sin when it is full grown it brings forth death." Temptation is an enticement for a person to an act that is evil, immoral, or unwise by promise of pleasure or gain. Whenever there is temptation or sin, the kingdom of darkness is ultimately behind it. Ephesians 6:12 says, "For our struggle is not against flesh and blood, but against the powers of this dark world and the spiritual forces of evil in the heavenly realms." The good news is that we can take every thought captive and make it obedient to Christ (1 Corinthians 10:5). 1 Corinthians 10:13 says, "No temptation has seized you except what is common to man. God is faithful, He will not let you be tempted beyond what you can bear. When you are tempted, He will provide a way of escape for you so you can stand up under it." Jesus understands how we feel because He suffered when He was tempted, and He is able to help those who are being tempted (Hebrews 2:18).

Read Matthew 4:1-11

v. 2, 3* Body- He was hungry after fasting 40 days and was tempted to turn stones into bread.

v. 6 * Soul- Made a choice to choose truth when tempted to prove *if* He was the Son of God.

v. 8, 9* Spirit- Temptation to worship Satan rather than God.

What principle of spiritual warfare can be learned from Jesus concerning what should be done when the attacks of the enemy come? (v. 4, 7, 10) Speaking Truth from the Word of God is a powerful weapon that will help us in our battles. After Jesus was victorious in the battle, He received blessing and anointing from God, He also was ministered to by angels. Jesus told His disciples in Luke 10:19 that, "He gave them authority to trample demonic powers and overcome ALL power of the enemy." The cross of Jesus sealed that victory for us, Jesus came to destroy the works of the devil according to 1 John 3:8. The blood that was shed on the cross is how Satan was defeated, it is powerful and life-giving! Leviticus 17:11 says, "For the life of the body is in its blood. I have given you the blood on the altar to purify you, making you right with the LORD. It is the blood, given in exchange for a life, which makes purification possible."

Here are just some of the provisions of the Blood of Jesus for the Christian:

Revelation 12:11—Overcomes the devil; John 6:54—Eternal life

Romans 5:9—Justified (saved from God's wrath)

Ephesians 1:7—Redemption (forgiveness of sins)

Colossians 1:20—Reconciled to God; 1 John 1:7—Purifies us from all sin

Hebrews 10:19—Enter into the Most Holy Place (God's presence)

How do I experience deliverance?

Romans 8:5, 6 says, "For those who live according to the flesh set their minds on the things of the flesh, but those who live according to the Spirit, the things of the Spirit. For to be carnally minded is death, but to be spiritually minded is life and peace."

1. Revelation—Pray and ask God where to start.
2. Repent—For holding on to the idols or sin in your life that He reveals.
3. Release—Commit everything to God, let go because He cares for you.
4. Renounce—Take away the legal right, cancel the contract you made with the demonic
5. Refill—Never leave an empty place, instead be filled with the Holy Spirit.
6. Restoration—Allow the healing of Jesus to renew your mind and transform you.
7. Reconciliation—The sweet unity of a friendship renewed- true communion.
8. Rejoice—Tell others what God has done … testimony is powerful!

SOUL-TIES

Just as a baby is connected to the umbilical cord for nourishment, we are connected to others for God's good purposes. However, when these relationships become unhealthy, they need to be cut. This is how we can continue to grow. The first thing God spoke to mankind was that it was not good to be alone. (Genesis 2:18). We are a three-in-one being, made in the image of God. The Father, Son, and Spirit are in perfect fellowship, and we are meant to experience unity with others. A soul-tie is when the soul is joined together, knitted (bonded) or a cleaving (hold fast to) occurs, in a sense the two become one, allowing life to be shared. The body of Christ is connected, and the life or energy of the Spirit is shared as brothers and sisters in the family of God.

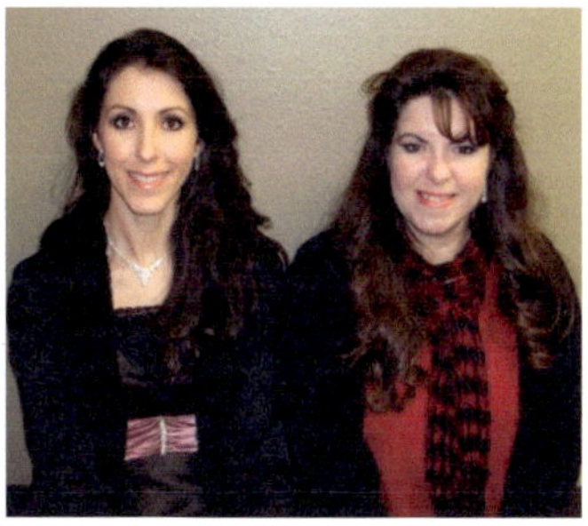

Above: Joanna Pixley and Jessica LaFavor are sisters, doulas, and the founders of Embracing Miracles.

Below: Courtney Dugstad served Next Chapter Ministries for over 10 years. She showed honor to all, fierce advocacy, and teamwork!

Soul:

- **Mind**—(thinking, reason, to know)
- **Emotion**—(feeling, to experience)
- **Will**—(decisions, choice, action)

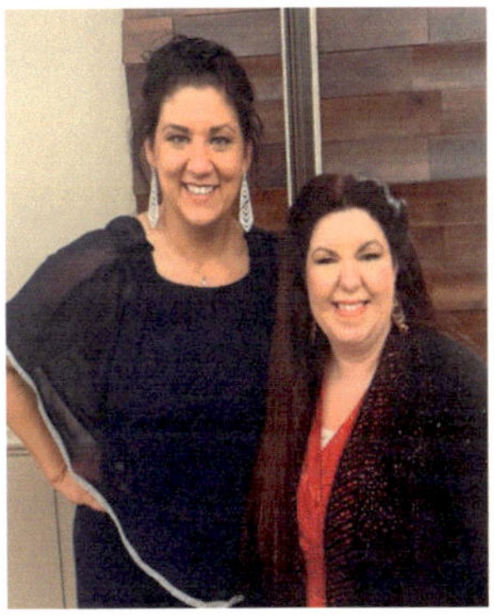

"Two are better than one because they have a good reward for their toil. For if they fall, one will lift his fellow. But woe to him who is alone when he falls and has not another to lift him up! Again, if two lie together, they keep warm, but how can one keep warm alone? And though a man might prevail against one who is alone, two will withstand him—a threefold cord is not quickly broken" (Ecclesiastes 4:9-12, NKJV). We are made for connection.

Godly Soul-ties

Husband and Wife—Genesis 2:24

God and you—Deuteronomy 10:20

Leader and People—2 Samuel 20:2

Parent and Child—Genesis 44:30

Friend to Friend—1 Samuel 18:1

Brothers and sisters—Colossians 3:12-15

Unhealthy Soul-ties

1. **Intellectual**—form when person becomes an idol, can't stop thinking about them. Loss of clear thinking, inability to make decisions, live in fantasy.

2. **Emotional**—form when your attachment to people, places, animals, and things are so important that you are unable or unwilling to give them up. Another way they form is when people have common feelings that are unbalanced or distorted (good or bad). Experiences fear, worry, anxiety.

3. **Sexual**—form at union, become negative when formed by sin. This can include adultery, rape, molestation, incest, pornography, masturbation, kissing.
   A spouse who is still connected in an unhealthy way to a mate that has died.

4. **Control**—form when someone tries to control us, or we give up our will.
   Co-dependency emerges in relationship, loss of individuality and identity.
   Self-confidence is based on what other, person thinks, says or does.
   One is unable to break away from the controlling person and assert their own will.

Ways a person can seek to control you are:
Excessive flattery, making decisions for you, over-protectiveness, being threatened by new decisions, financial manipulation, being super-spiritual (holy than thou attitude).
May experience anger, resentment, helplessness, and have no boundaries in place.

Unhealthy soul-ties can cause the loss of:
Good health, the ability to really love others, personal freedom, spiritual liberty, and protection. Closeness to the Lord and hearing Him. To prevent unhealthy soul ties from forming: Establish strong soul-ties with God. This means committing all your soul (mind, emotion, will) to God and be willing to submit to Him.

Resist the Devil and know where you stand. Establish firm boundaries in relationships, put the Cross of Christ in the middle of all relationships. This way you will be connected through the truth; but not bound to them. Learn who you are in Christ, find your identity.

Finally, have a standard of purity in place. Blessed is the man that endures temptation; for when he is tried, he shall receive the crown of life, which the Lord has promised to those who love Him (James 1:12).

Breaking Soul-Ties Prayer:

Thank you, Lord, for revealing to me this block in our relationship. Father God, I repent for allowing this unhealthy soul tie of (name sin).

I repent of the sin of idolatry, of allowing this relationship to become a hindrance in my life with you. I forgive (the person with whom the soul tie was made) for their part in making and strengthening this unhealthy soul tie.

I break this soul tie in the Name of Jesus and renounce every unholy part of the bond. I break any hold that the demonic has in this soul tie and send them to the feet of the Lord Jesus.

I call back every emotion, thought, and part of the will that was given to (__________) and I give back every emotion, thought, and part of the will that was imparted.

Thank you, Lord, for your healing of my mind, will, and emotions and the wholeness that you bring. In Jesus Name Amen!

Steps to Freedom: 2 Timothy 2:20-26

- We choose to be a vessel of honor or dishonor
- Cleanse ourselves from sin, to be sanctified; prepared for good purposes
- Flee youthful lusts and pursue: Righteousness, Faith, Love, Peace
- Avoid foolish arguments, knowing that they cause strife.
- Must not quarrel, but be gentle, able to teach, patient
- Correct those in opposition, pray that God will grant them repentance
- Know the truth, come to our senses—recover ourselves from the trap.

REDEMPTION OF THE LORD'S CHOSEN: STEPS TO SALVATION

Over the course of my time at the *Rochester Outreach Center*, there was a small group of people, both men and women who had a heart to see the physical and spiritual needs of people being met in their local community. This included women and families be met through doula services and for all who came to the ROC to see the love of Jesus! This is where the first Embracing Miracles office was and so much planning, prayer and preparation took place for doula training and *Women of Strength* events.

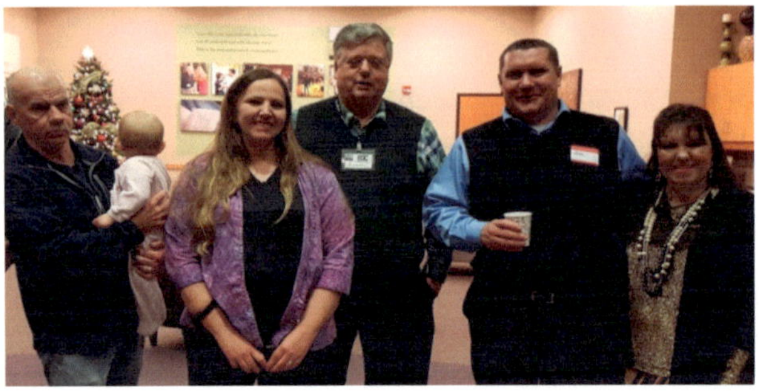

ROC Team- Robert and Jen Clanton, Rev. Dale DePeel, Nate Augeson, Jessica LaFavor, Melodie Schwartz, Shay Jones, and Nancy Ventura.

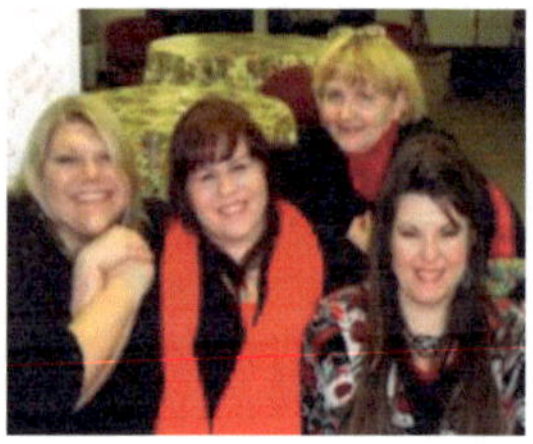

Redemption was God's plan of restoration (**salvation**) from the beginning for mankind (Ephesians 1:4-7). Redemption (**setting free by payment**) is the recovery of that which was lost through sin- breaking God's law, the payment for sin is death. We have all broken God's law and cannot be good enough to save ourselves. For all have sinned and fallen short of the glory (**standard**) of God. (Romans 3:23). Just take the Ten Commandments for example (Exodus 20: 3-17). Who can really claim that they have kept God's standard for righteousness? The first people who were ever created Adam and Eve disobeyed God; thus, the curse of sin and death entered the world. Their initial response was to hide and cover their own sin.

However, God is a righteous judge. So, justice had to be served, a sacrifice had to be made. God Himself covered them with animal skins (Genesis 3:21). What had to happen to the animal? It had to die. The skins covered their bodies, and the blood covered their sin. The Bible makes it very clear that there is no forgiveness of sins, without the shedding of blood (Hebrews 9:22). Jesus is called the Lamb of God who takes away the sins of the world. (John 1:29).

God (**Our Heavenly Father**) loved the world so much that He gave His one and only Son, so that everyone who believes in Him will not perish but have eternal life (John 3:16). This means that Jesus took the punishment that we deserved; He paid the price. It was the only way to satisfy God's anger towards sin.

For the wages (**what we earn**) of sin (**breaking God's law**) is death, but the gift of God is eternal life (**living with God forever in Heaven**) through Jesus Christ our Lord. (Romans 6:23). We can never be good enough to earn salvation. You are saved by grace (God's love) through faith (**belief**), not of yourselves, it is the gift of God. Not of works, so no one can boast about it (Ephesians 2:8-9). If you confess (**agree**) with your mouth the Lord Jesus and believe in your heart that God raised Him from the dead, you will be saved. (Romans 10:9-10; Matthew 25:34). If someone is not saved from God's wrath (**anger**) then he is destined to eternal punishment and death in hell. (Romans 2:5-6; 2 Thessalonians 1:8-9; Matthew 25:46).

This is not God's heart ... 2 Peter 3:9 says, "The Lord isn't being slow about His promise (**to come back**), as some think. No, he is being patient for your sake. He does not want anyone to be destroyed but wants everyone to repent." Sin always causes separation from God. Isaiah 59:2.

A **Revelation** of who God is brings **Repentance**, leading to **Reconciliation** of **Relationship** ...

Revelation: <u>Making something known in a dramatic way, spiritual knowledge</u>

*__God__ is our Creator and has been revealed through His creation to display His Glory. (Romans 1:16-25).

*In the beginning was the Word, the revelation of **Jesus** the light of the world. (John 1:1-5; 11-14).

* The plan of salvation has been revealed and the **Holy Spirit** is given to us. (Ephesians 1:9-14).

Repentance: <u>To change one's mind, Turn away from sin- to God, Remorse for actions</u>

*God draws us first; Godly sorrow produces repentance leading to salvation. (John 6:44, 2 Corinthians 7:10).

* If wicked people turn from their wickedness and do what is right, they will live. (Ezekiel 18:23-32)

*Jesus said to Repent and believe in the Gospel because the Kingdom of God is near. (Mark 1:15).

Reconciliation: Restoration; bringing together again, making peace, friendship (Ephesians 2:13-16).

*God showed His love by sending Jesus to die for us while we were still sinners. (Romans 5:1-11).

*We go from darkness to light; Jesus made peace through the blood of His cross. (Colossians 1:12-21).

*In Christ you are a new person, given a message of reconciliation for others. (2 Corinthians 5:17-20).

Relationship: Connection, intimacy—closeness, working together, unity—and family

*Jesus is the Way, the Truth, and the Life—no one comes to God except through Christ. (John 14:6).

*Faith and hope are in God and His Word; we must grow in Him and follow. (1 Peter 1:3-2:6; John 10:27).

* As children of God, we have His love and Spirit in us. (1 John 3:1-3, 16-24).

CHAPTER 12

POSTPARTUM TIME: RECOVERY

PHYSICAL RECOVERY

a.) Healing

In the weeks after having a new baby, it can be a time of adjustment for everyone. Depending on the kind of birth it was, there may be physical healing. If the birth experience did not meet expectations, there may also be emotional healing as well. The mother is often sleep-deprived and has a lot of hormone changes going on in her body. Postpartum depression affects some women and can become serious. During the postpartum visit, I do an emotional check-in and we discuss any warning signs that may be affecting the mother. It is important to be aware of certain moods and emotional changes that may occur and seek medical help if required. Having a postpartum doula can help at home in the time after delivery. Her role is to be of service in various ways including light cleaning, cooking, laundry, errands, getting information, goal setting, and helping with the care of other children as well as the new baby and a listening ear.

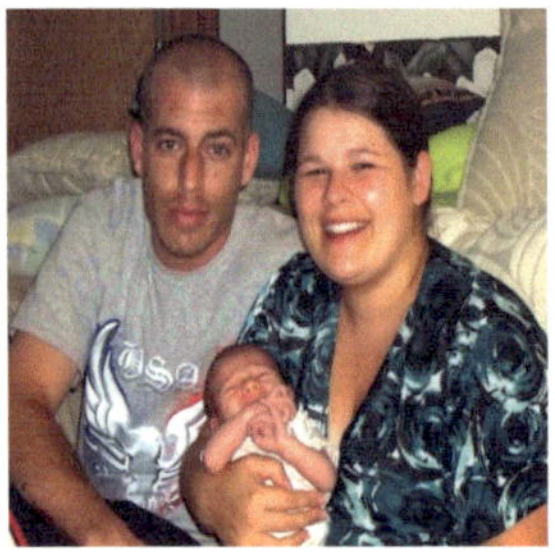

Drew and Leah with baby Riley after a long labor ending in a C-section. She had a lot of back labor. Drew applied counter pressure and we did a lot of moving through her labor, which helped. However, exhaustion became a component in their decision to have surgery and meet their son.

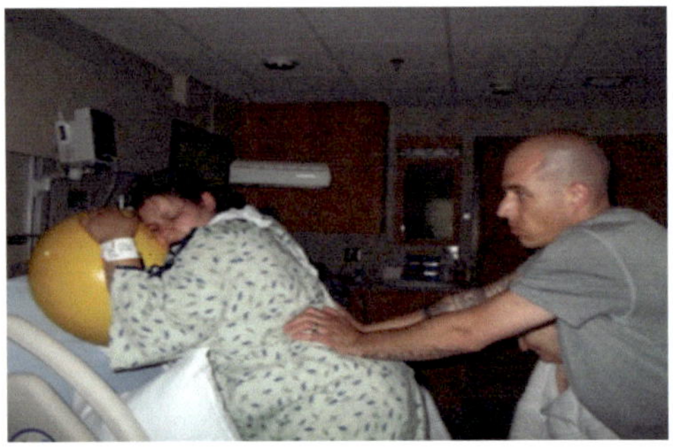

b.) Bonding

The hour after delivery is a very special time. This is when the chemistry between mother and baby is established. Skin-to-skin contact and feeding the baby encourages bonding. Even fathers who engage in skin-to-skin with their babies notice more of a connection than fathers who do not. It is important to have an atmosphere that is undisrupted and quiet. Visitors can wait until the new family has a chance to get to know each other first. This is a most precious, intimate time.

Our philosophy is "Love at birth, love for life."

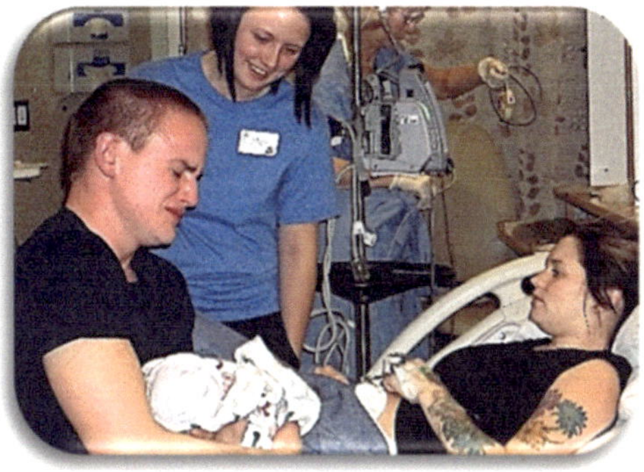

Eden had a beautiful labor with her daughter Eve. She had the support of her sister-in-law Faith as well as her husband, Jonah. He is enveloped in the emotion of holding their baby girl for the first time!

c.) Resting

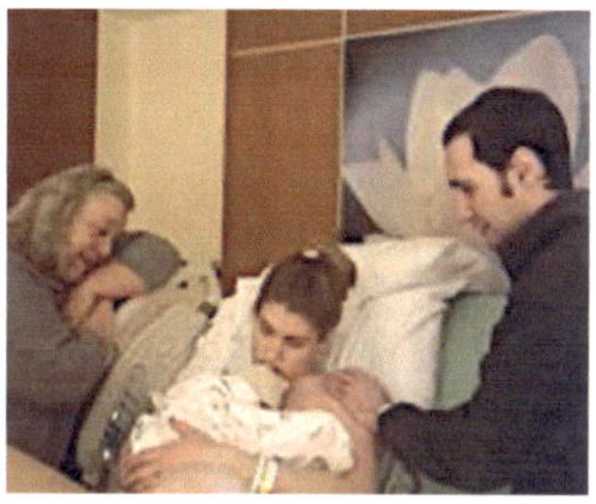

Emily and Christian relax now that the hard work is done. Their daughter Claire is finally here! Grandma Judi was there to witness this wonderful birth and will be instrumental in helping when they get home.

Being able to balance the responsibilities of motherhood can leave finding enough time to rest quite a challenge. It is important for moms to realize that resting while the baby rests is essential to her health, this is a part of the healing process. The more rested and relaxed a woman is, the easier it is to have a proper perspective. When other children are already present, this is when a friend, neighbor, family, or doula can be very helpful. It is a good idea to form a postpartum plan while you are doing a birth plan. To answer the following questions such as, who will cook, clean, pay bills, and so on, can help alleviate stress later.

RESILIENCY (ANNIE AND MATT'S STORY)

Annie and I met while working for a local nonprofit organization, Next Chapter Ministries in Rochester, MN. We would become friends, going from being co-workers to being co-laborers. In our job, we served those who had been impacted by the cycle of incarceration and the mission was to see God's restoration in their lives. We knew the value of resiliency.

On January 10th Annie was waiting for me as I arrived at 9:30 am, and we prayed together before she took her Castor oil drink to begin the at-home induction. Her midwife suggested this because her liver enzymes were elevated. At 11 am Annie took a nap; she was feeling pretty good about everything. Matt had been vacuuming since I got there and was nesting even more than Annie. They are so excited about this baby's new arrival. 12:30 pm Annie is starting to feel nauseous she's going to drink some tea. At 1:00 pm there was some loose stool. At 2:00 pm she began feeling crampy. At 3:00 pm she took the second shot. We used the rebozo to do some abdominal lifts to relieve the pressure. 3:30 pm, we used the rebozo and the birth ball. It was a very peaceful day we had worship music on, and we did art at the kitchen table. I also made sure that Annie and Matt were eating throughout the day.

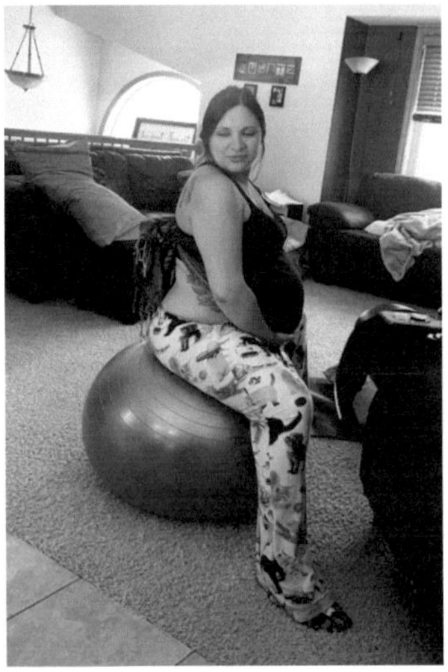

4:00 pm Annie was doing the mile circuit and then the ball circuit and then the mile circuit again. As she was stretching and releasing her breath, there were more contractions. At 4:30 pm there was some early labor. By 6:00 pm she was resting on the yoga mat and had a smoothie. Around 6:42 pm there was some bloody show.

7:00 pm the waves are getting more intense and closer together, shortly thereafter, we texted the birth team. By 7:30 pm Matt was getting the pool ready, and Annie was in the rocking chair breathing. The midwife team was on their way and Grandma Jeanette (Annie's mom) was there with the girls. 8:45 pm there's more standing and rocking. Matt and Annie are connecting a lot more now, and Ivy the midwife's assistant arrived. Annie cleaned herself up after vomiting and felt much better! By 9:05 pm Terry the hypnobirthing doula is also here and by 9:20 pm Meg her midwife arrives. Terry is rubbing Annie's back as she stands through contractions.

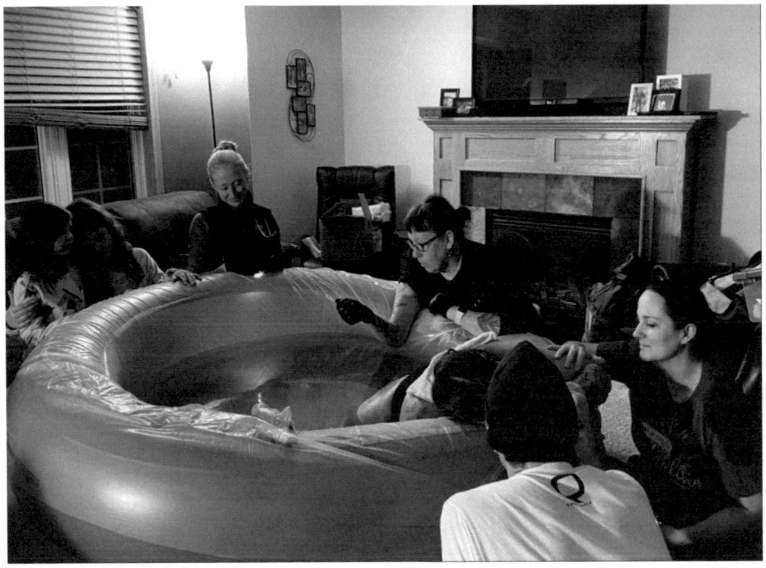

At 9:30 pm Meg checks Annie and she is 80% effaced and 5 centimeters dilated. At 9:45 pm, Annie got into the birth tub and only Terry and Matt stayed upstairs. Around 10:30 pm labor was becoming more intense. At 10:35 pm Annie's water broke, and she began to feel very pushy. The midwives came up from downstairs and we collected the girls from their room with their grandma and asked them to come to join us in the living room it was then that Annie began to push. A sweet baby girl arrived through water birth at 10:51 pm (6.15 lbs.).

After a few moments of joyful welcoming, we helped Annie out of the pool and into her bedroom to deliver the placenta. Annie was not having the normal afterbirth pains, but she was enjoying her baby and after a few moments we decided to let Matt have some skin-to-skin with her while we concentrated on the delivery of the placenta. Meg the midwife and her assistant Ivy decided to give a shot of Pitocin to Annie to help the process along. We then went into the bathroom for her to sit on the toilet and see if that would help. I was holding the scissors because by then the midwife had cut the baby's cord. We sat for a long while and we were just reminiscing about how perfect everything had gone with the birth.

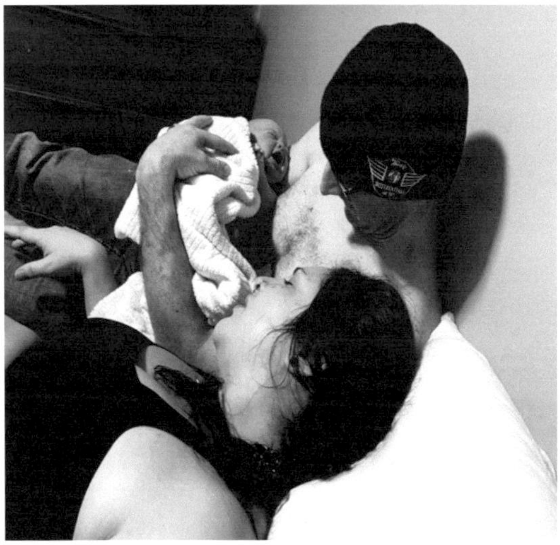

We went back out and the midwives had a birth stool ready for Annie to sit on so Matt got behind her and she put the baby to breast, and we were hoping the placenta would just naturally deliver but it didn't. They gave Annie another shot of Pitocin, and we were reaching about an hour postpartum by this time.

Suddenly Annie's eyes went glassy, and her head began to shake ever so slightly we knew Annie was going into shock the midwife asked for me to call 911 so I did (11:42 pm). As we were on the phone with the paramedics on their way, we were explaining to the dispatcher exactly what the events were. Annie's face turned colors and she began to lose consciousness. The ambulance was on its way, and everybody stayed calm. I of course was saying a silent prayer of peace and protection not only for Annie but for everyone in the room, for the girls, and for Grandma as well. The paramedics arrived very shortly thereafter, and it took a long while for them to get everything situated for Annie to go to the hospital. I took the baby, and I got her dressed in her first outfit, a red checker flannel. Then I let Jeanette hold her before I ran her out to where Annie was getting ready to go to the hospital in the ambulance. She was accompanied by Meg the midwife and Matt her husband. I went back in the house and prayed with the girls, Terry, and Ivy. They stayed back to do the clean-up from birth.

I arrived at the hospital at 12:45 am. Annie was in surgery by the time I got there. Nurses were talking about it as I approached the desk, and I was asked to sit in the waiting area. Fortunately, Meg texted me to fill me in on what was happening. She came and brought me to the room where they were. Apparently, the hospital staff tried to manually deliver the placenta and her uterus had ruptured.

So, I sat with Meg the midwife, Matt, and miss Evelyn Jean who had just come into this world. The surgeon came in at about 1:15 am and said that Annie was in very serious condition and that they were doing everything they could to save her life but that they might very well have to do a hysterectomy, she had placenta accreta.

In the meanwhile, the little baby was hungry and so we gave her a bottle of formula and we all just stayed calm in prayerful mode. We decided to try to look for some donor milk so that Evelyn could have breast milk while Annie was in recovery. Ivy was still breastfeeding and was good enough to pump some milk and brought to the hospital when she picked up Meg, they left around 3:00 am. The surgery was finished at about 3:15 am, they did end up doing a hysterectomy on Annie and give her blood transfusions to strengthen her after surgery.

Once Annie was in the ICU, Matt and the baby girl accompanied her up there and that's where they spent the night. I left at about 3:45 am and was so happy to hear from Annie in the morning! She was conscious and understood what had happened to her the night before. We were able to process a little bit of this birth experience a week later. Baby Evelyn was precious and perfect, breastfeeding wonderfully. Mom and baby are doing great! Annie knows that there is going to be a time when she's got to process some of what happened, but she knows that she will have the resilience to do so, and she has her strength and faith rooted in God.

She was very grateful for the entire birth team and she and Matt have a journey of wonderful parenting ahead of them. I'm very thankful for the incredible birth team Annie had and how we all worked together in an amazing way during this experience. My prayer was that Annie would have a quick recovery and she would have peaceful rest in the weeks following her delivery. It's time to just spend time getting used to this little girl and focus on the family's transition. I am so incredibly grateful and honored that I could be in this place of holding spiritual space and peace for this family while this little baby entered the world.

SPIRITUAL RECOVERY

a.) Faith-based

When we first enter into the new life of Christ, there is a process of the old passing away and the new coming, according to 2 Corinthians 5:17. The Word goes further by saying, "that you put off, concerning your former conduct, the old man which grows corrupt according to the deceitful lusts, and be renewed in the spirit of your mind, and that you put on the new man which was created according to God, in true righteousness and holiness." (Ephesians 4:22-24 NKJV). Sometimes our old conduct is difficult to overcome. There are many good tools to help us in our struggles. Some of these tools may include prayer, music, a mantra, or Scripture aloud, finding a support group, having an accountability partner, affirmations, or working through a 12-step program. The reality is that we have victory through the power of the Spirit.

A cool "Hippie Chick" named Sheri became my first sponsor when I got out of drug and alcohol treatment and began attending recovery meetings. I was living in a halfway house, and she taught me the value of having sober fun! We have celebrated almost 30 years in recovery and friendship. When I was her doula for her daughter Daisy years ago, she gave me the tag line- "Doulafavor".

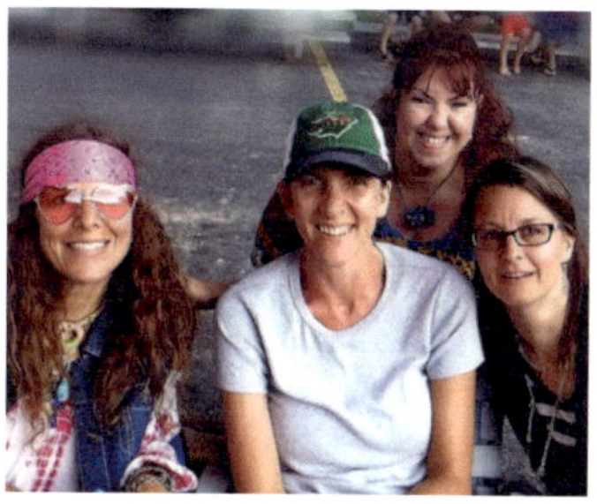

Sheri, Monica, Jessica, and Julie all met through the doors of recovery and found freedom, friendship and faith that have lasted a lifetime!

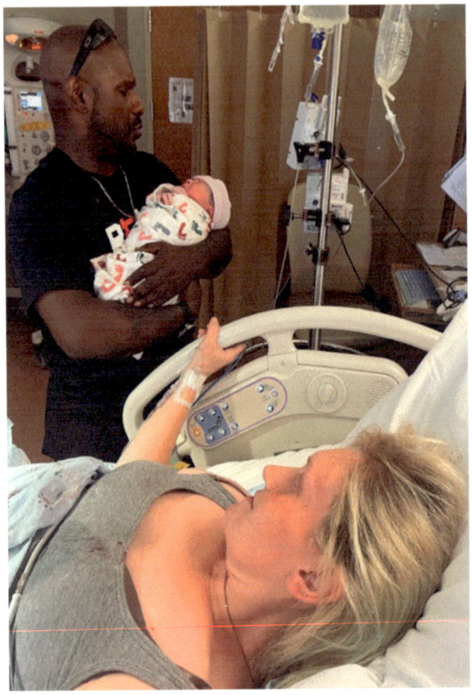

Kip and Kalie are a couple who are in recovery from addiction. Faith-based recovery plays a part in establishing a new life of freedom. Their daughter Kenzleigh symbolizes all they have worked so hard for. Transformation is a process that takes time but is well worth it!

I met Kalie while she was incarcerated, and we began our relationship there. She had other children that she did not have custody of because of her former lifestyle. However, although CPS was involved, Kalie and Kip were both determined to see a different outcome for their daughter.

After taking responsibility and availing themselves of the support network they had, they did all that was not only required but wanted by them to accomplish the goal of parenthood. Their case was eventually closed, and they were able to go forward as a family!

b.) Fellowship

The incredible nature of God is very telling in that He is one God, but a fellowship. of three persons. We are created for connection with a purpose. When we have children and add to our families, this is where fellowship starts. However, when we become Christians, there is the fellowship of believers. Let us consider how we may spur one another on toward love and good deeds, not giving up meeting together, as some are in the habit of doing but encouraging one another (Hebrews 10:24-25 NIV). This gives us the opportunity to be strengthened in the Body of Christ. We must continue steadfastly in the apostles' doctrine and fellowship, in the breaking of bread, and in prayers." (Acts 2:42 NKJV).

c.) Peace

The experience after we receive Jesus as Lord is knowing Him as the Prince of Peace. In John 14:27, Jesus promises this, "**Peace** I leave with you, My **peace** I give to you; not as the world gives do I give to you. Let not your heart be troubled, neither let it be afraid…and the **peace** of God, which surpasses all understanding, will guard your hearts and minds through Christ Jesus (Philippians 4:17). God's peace enables us to go through hardships and suffering and temptation knowing that we are never alone,

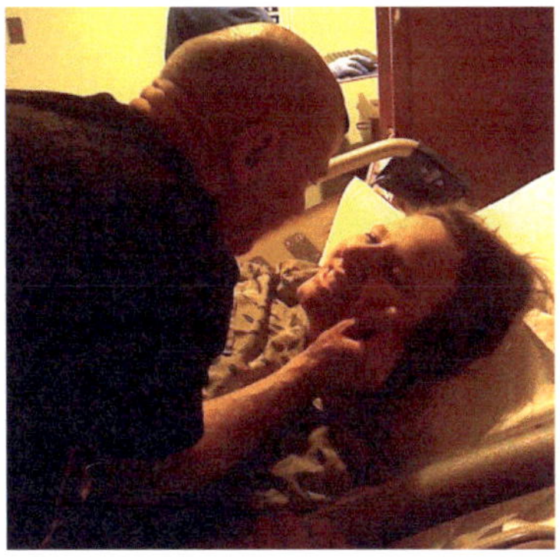

the presence of God is our peace. As we learn to flow in the peace that we have, our example can clearly be seen by the world. 1Thessolonians 5:23 reminds us, "Now may the God of **peace** Himself sanctify you completely; and may your whole spirit, soul, and body be preserved blameless at the coming of our Lord Jesus Christ." (NKJV).

Robert and Jen Clanton illuminating the peace of God during the labor of their daughter Abigail.

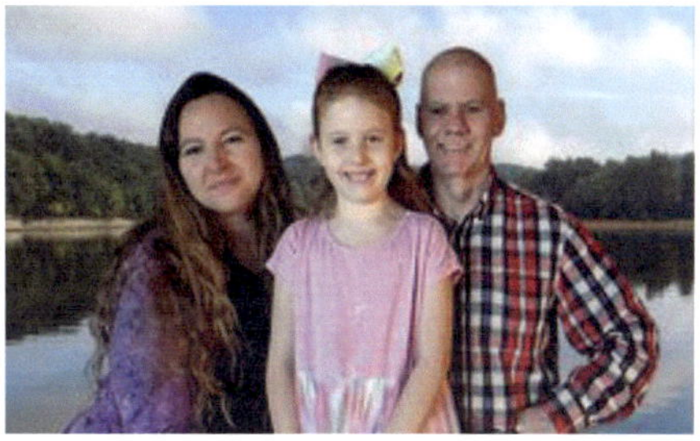

Growing up, my Uncle Robert always brought a sense of peace whenever he was in my life. He has been a co-laborer of the Grateful Life team as Captain of the Intercessory prayer team since its inception; he received healing, deliverance and, eventually ministry training through *Cleansing Streams Ministries.* As we waited together for the promises of God to come to fulfillment, much ministry took place! His beautiful wife Jen was brought into our lives as we all served together at the Rochester Outreach Center. She is such a treasure and one of the biggest advocates for the care of others! She attended a DONA doula training as well as the Heart of a Doula workshop through Grateful Life and we had the honor of walking alongside a few wonderful families in birth work and bringing spiritual new life during *Women of Strength* events. This power couple has the heart to see the truth of God's Spirit and Word breathe life into the lost and bring hope to the broken.

CHAPTER 13

MOTHER AND NEWBORN CARE

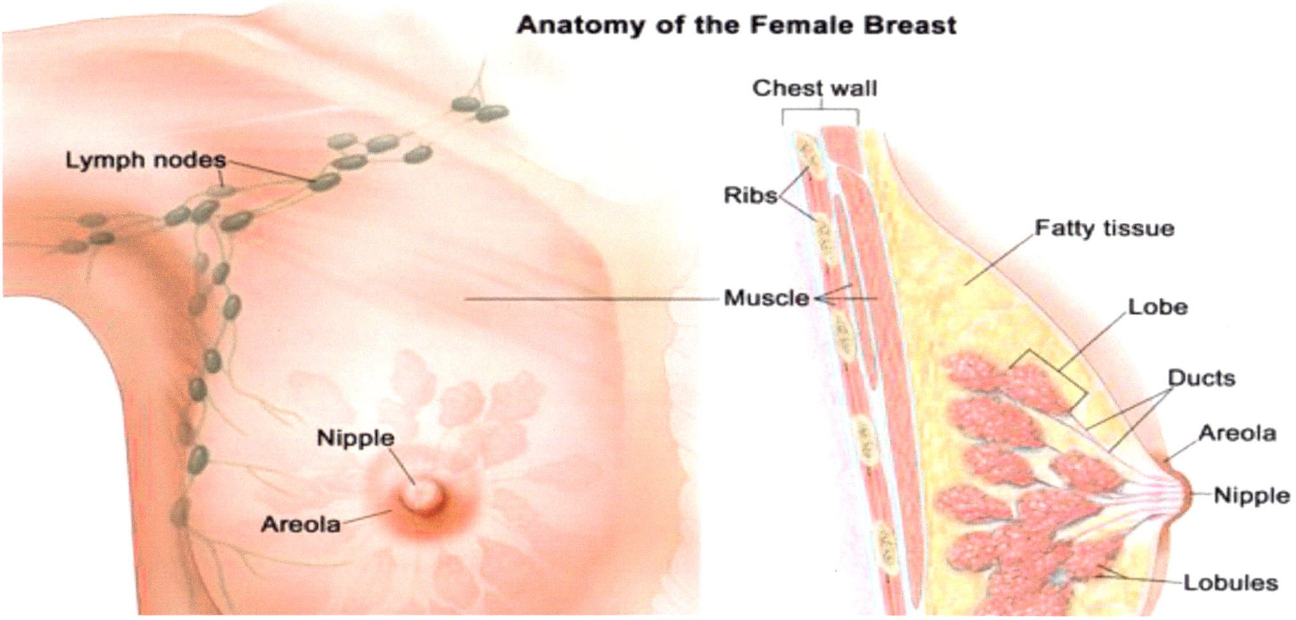

PHYSICAL HEALTH

a.) Breastfeeding

God designed a woman's body not only to conceive and carry a child but to nourish that child as well. Mother's milk is a novelty in the body, just as it is needed for a newborn and growing baby. During pregnancy, the physical changes begin in preparation for milk production. The intricate physiology of breastfeeding includes these four hormones that help your breasts make milk: **estrogen, progesterone, prolactin,** and **oxytocin.** The mother's body naturally knows how to help her breasts make milk. **Estrogen** and **progesterone** are released by the placenta during pregnancy. Their two main functions are to increase the size and number of milk ducts in your breasts. They also keep your body from making a large quantity of breast milk until after your baby is born. Once your baby and the placenta are delivered, these hormones decrease, which signals your body that it is time to make milk. After the birth of your baby, prolactin levels increase. Every time you breastfeed or pump, your body releases prolactin. With each release, your body makes and stores more milk in the breast alveoli. If the level of this hormone gets too low, your milk supply will decrease. Therefore, it is important to breastfeed or pump right after delivery and regularly after that.

Oxytocin releases milk from your breasts. When your baby (or breast pump) begins to suck and draw your nipple into her mouth, this hormone is released. Milk is squeezed out of the alveoli, into the ducts and out of your nipple, into your baby's mouth. This process is called letdown, a tingling sensation in the breast before or during a feeding. Other signs may include:

1. Milk flowing from her breasts when she thinks of the baby or hears him crying.
2. Slow deep sucks and swallowing, which shows that milk is flowing into his mouth.
3. Uterine pain or a flow of blood from the uterus.
4. Being thirsty during a feeding. It is extremely important to be well-hydrated.

The main reflexes of a baby are **rooting** (finding), **suckling** (filling), and s**wallowing** (drinking). When supporting a mother and baby in the beginning of breastfeeding, it is important to know about these reflexes. It is so important for the baby to have a good latch, remember that the baby is suckling from the breast, not from the nipple. Try different positions until you find something that works for the mother and baby.

Some early difficulties which may arise include:

- sore nipples/poor latch
- flat/inverted nipples
- refusal to latch
- engorgement/plugged ducts/mastitis breast pain
- fatigue
- infant crying/sleeping

Resources are available for mothers who are having trouble breastfeeding, such as nurses, doulas, and lactation consultants. Colostrum is the clear, yellowish liquid produced in the first few days after birth. It is high in protein, east to digest and rich in immunities. As doulas, part of what we teach is the benefit of breastfeeding and help support the mother as she learns this skill. The complexity of breastfeeding is completely in line with the order that God created the entire universe to function in, it's absolutely amazing!

b.) Nutrition

Food is the fuel for the body. The value of proper nutrition and health during pregnancy, labor and the postpartum period cannot be underestimated. Here is a list to start with:

- soups saltine crackers graham crackers fruits bananas
- jello pasta honey sticks toast broth
- yogurt herbal tea white grape juice apple juice rice
- cereal noodles cooked cereals popsicles applesauce
- scrambled or boiled egg pudding granola trail mix

Fathers are not the ones in labor; however, it is important not to forget them. All of the physiological changes that occur during childbirth may inhibit some women from feeling hungry, but that is not the case with dads. No one wants to see a father faint because his blood sugar drops. So, by all means, remind them to bring some snacks for themselves. If you are attending a hospital birth, make sure to go over helpful tips with your clients regarding food options—knowing cafeteria hours, money for vending machines, eating before leaving home.

Being well-hydrated is not only important in pregnancy, but also in labor and beyond. A mother's body is working physically hard and using a lot of energy. Make sure to remind laboring women to take drinks after every few contractions. Some hospitals start an IV so that dehydration does not occur. Every time a woman needs to urinate during labor, the better. This puts her pelvis in a great position to give birth, so bring on the fluids!

How about after the baby comes? Well to make breast milk, one needs enough hydration. So, make sure that mom has a tall glass of juice, herbal tea, or water every time she nurses. Steps to a healthy lifestyle during pregnancy: Physical activity and exercise, a variety of nutritious foods, vitamins and supplements, and self-care.

c.) Baby Language

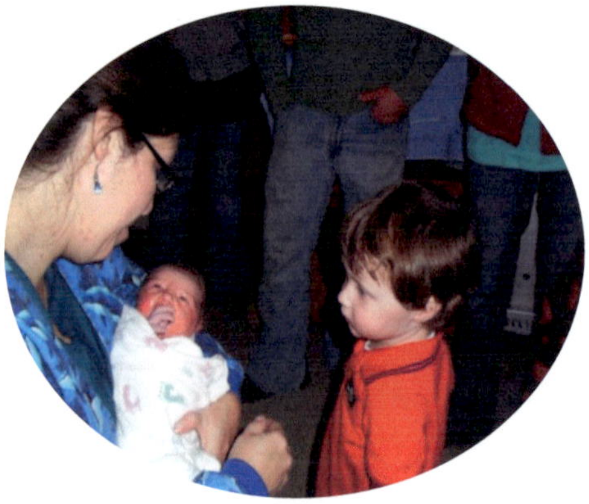

Being able to understand your new baby is essential for meeting his or her needs. Just as non-verbal communication can be learned, so can the different cries and sounds of an infant. Sometimes a baby needs to be fed or changed, other times the baby needs to be burped or moved around. One can begin listening to the various types of communication as soon as the baby is born. Learning the sounds and cues of a baby will enable a parent to build security and trust in the life of their child as the journey of parenthood continues. It is a good option for parents to avail themselves of the many good resources and tools to learn more about understanding their baby language.
We can help parents determine how to listen to their baby's cues.

Ask: "Does your baby need to be fed, burped, moved, changed, or maybe held?"

As they get to know the sounds of the baby, they will begin to understand what he or she needs.

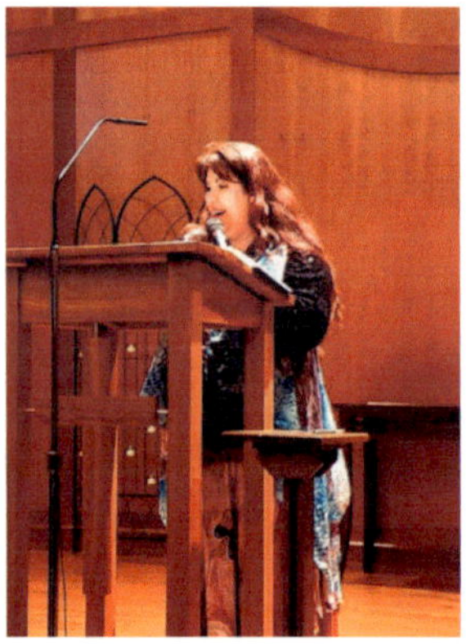

SPIRITUAL HEALTH

a.) Pure Milk of the Word

2 Peter 2:2 says, "Like newborn infants, long for the pure spiritual milk, that by it you may grow up into salvation" (ESV). After a baby is born, even within the very first hour, it is already using instinctual behaviors that God created, to nourish him or herself. When we are born again, as new Christians, it becomes natural to hunger and wants to be filled with the Word of God. However, there is a growing process, babies are only ready for milk, not other food. 1 Corinthians 3:1-2 tells us that, "I could not address you as spiritual people, but as people of the flesh, as infants in Christ. I fed you with milk, not solid food, for you were not ready for it. And even now you are not yet ready" …

For though by this time, you ought to be teachers, you need someone to teach you again the basic principles of the oracles of God. You need milk, not solid food, for everyone who lives on milk is unskilled in the word of righteousness since he is a child. But solid food is for the mature, for those who have their powers of discernment trained by constant practice to distinguish good from evil. (Hebrews 5:12-14, ESV) May each one of us continue to mature and be nourished with the pure spiritual milk of the Word of God and grow into the deeper truths that God has for us.

b.) Communion

Part of spiritual growth is being a part of a family. Just as a child is born into a family to be loved, nurtured, held accountable, and continue to mature, so it is in the body of Christ. His divine power has granted to us all things that pertain to life and godliness, through the knowledge of him who called us to his own glory and excellence, by which he has granted to us his precious and very great promises, so that through them you may become partakers of the divine nature, having escaped from the corruption that is in the world… (2 Peter 1:3,4 ESV).

In John 17, Jesus prays for us saying, **[21] "I pray that they will all be one, just as you and I are one**—as you are in me, Father, and I am in you … May they experience such perfect unity that the world will know that you sent me and that you love them as much as you love me." Jesus desires us to be just as close as He is with His Father. To have communion with the Lord is to experience perfect unity in the spirit. When we as Christians celebrate Communion or the *Lord's Table*, we are remembering the promises and sacrifice of Jesus. Not only that but also that we are His bride whom He is coming back for!

c.) Hearing God's Voice

Just as new parents learn to listen to the sounds of their baby, as new spiritual babes, we listen to the voice of God. If we can't "hear" (feel, sense, experience) God clearly, we become open to deception. In John chapter 10:27-28, Jesus gives this encouragement, "My sheep hear my voice, and I know them, and they follow me. I give them eternal life, and they will never perish, and no one will snatch them out of my hand." (ESV). Hearing the voice of God is essential for avoiding sin, getting direction for our life, and having daily peace. Just as there are various cries of a baby, there are also many ways that God speaks to us. *And your ears shall hear a word behind you, saying, "This is the way, walk in it ..."* (Isaiah 30:21 ESV). Prayer is a pathway not only for communion with God in our communication but also a way to hear Him clearly as well. We were created to hear God through our spirit, not our soul. As we learn to walk in the spirit and submit to the Lord's leading, we no longer hear God through the filter of our soul (mind-what we think, will-what we want, and emotions- how we feel).

The Holy Spirit reveals the truth to us. John 16:13 says, "When the Spirit of truth comes, He will guide you into all the truth, for he will not speak on his own authority but whatever he hears he will speak, and he will declare to you the things that are to come ... For the word of God is living and active, sharper than any two-edged sword, piercing to the division of soul and of spirit, of joints and of marrow, and discerning the thoughts and intentions of the heart." (Hebrews 4:12, ESV). All Scripture is breathed out by God and profitable for teaching, reproof, correction, and training in righteousness, that the man of God may be completely equipped for every good wor*k.* (2 Timothy 3:16-17, ESV).

God sometimes will speak to us in visions and dreams as well ... Acts 2:17 says, "In the last days, God says, I will pour out my Spirit on all people. Your sons **and** daughters will prophesy, your young men will see **visions**, your old men will dream **dreams**." No matter how God chooses to speak to us, it will bring us hope; we should be ready to hear Him. Like a good father, He is always ready to hear us.

PHYSICAL EXERCISE

a.) Daily

Exercise is part of ongoing good health for new mothers. Some of the benefits include: More energy, improves mood, increased focus, weight loss, decreased risk of certain diseases, better sleep, helps to relieve stress and anxiety, and it can be lots of fun. A good goal for exercise is at least 30 minutes daily. One can walk, bike, run, dance, do aerobics, hike, swim, or do anything that gets you moving! Setting a regular time to exercise every day and keeping a log can help it become a habit.

b.) Training

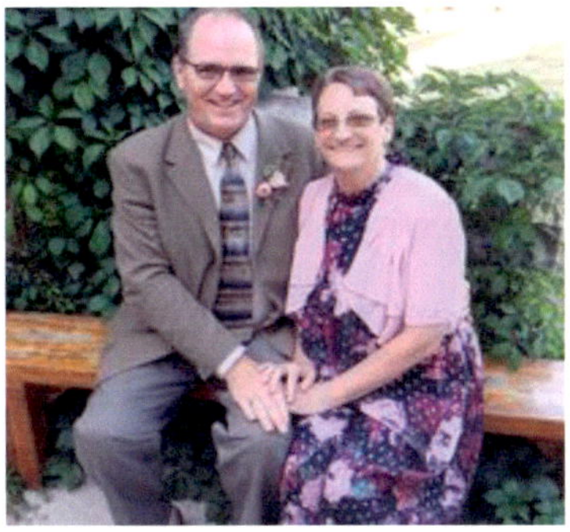

The Bible speaks of the importance of exercise and godly training in 1 Timothy 4:6-8 when it says … "Be a good servant of Christ Jesus, being trained in the words of the faith and of the good doctrine that you have followed. Have nothing to do with irreverent, silly myths. Rather train yourself for godliness; for physical training is of some value, but godliness has value for all things, holding promise for both the present life and the life to come." 2 Timothy 2:5 goes on to say, "An athlete is not crowned unless he competes according to the rules." Anyone who has ever been in competition knows just how much hard work and training it takes to win! When God gives the gift of children, He expects parents to train them as Proverbs 22:6 says, "Train up a child in the way he should go; even when he is old, he will not depart from it."

God is faithful in giving us the training we need to accomplish His purposes and we train our own children for God's glory.

TAC CENTER TRAIN A CHILD
The real **hope** for **change** is how we **raise** them.

Rev. Johann and Stephanie Marsland have been an example of true hospitality in word and deed. Their heart for education led them to start a Christian school to provide ministry and parent partnerships.

c.) Discipline

Being a disciplined person is very difficult in this day and age. We are used to immediate gratification and entitlement. However, being diligent in exercise after a new baby will pay off! Start a routine, and maybe include a friend who can keep you accountable. You should start off slow and warm up first before exercise.

Spiritual discipline is something that new believers need, just as a mother needs physical discipline. *"Don't you realize that in a race everyone runs, but only one person gets the prize? So, run to win! All athletes are disciplined in their training. They do it to win a prize that will fade away, but we do it for an eternal prize. So, I run with purpose in every step. I am not just shadowboxing. I discipline my body like an athlete, training it to do what it should. Otherwise, I fear that after preaching to others I might be disqualified."* (1 Corinthians 9:24-27, NLT).

SPIRITUAL EXERCISE

a.) Bible Study

We, like Joshua, need to take what God says to heart in Joshua 1:8, *and* "**Study this Book** of Instruction continually**. Meditate on it** day and night so you will be sure to **obey** everything written in it. Only then will you prosper and succeed in all you do." Our work as Doulas depends on having the right instructions for whom we are serving at any given moment. As our relationship with Christ grows, we must be like the Bereans who … "Received the word with all readiness and **searched the Scriptures daily** *to find out* whether these things were so." (Acts 17:11, NKJV). Jesus said, "Man shall not live on bread alone, but on **every word** that comes from the mouth of God." (Matthew 4:4, NIV). Reading and meditating on Scripture is vital for spiritual health. I will **study** your commandments and **reflect** on your ways. (Psalm 119:15, NLT).

b.) Prayer

As a part of a Christian's spiritual exercise, prayer must be the center of it all. Prayer is powerful and changes things! 2 Chronicles 7:14 says, "Then if my people who are called by my name will humble themselves and **pray** and seek my face and turn from their wicked ways, I will hear from heaven and will forgive their sins and restore their land." Jesus, Himself often withdrew to the wilderness for **prayer** and taught His disciples how to pray in Matthew 6:9-13.

"Our Father in heaven, your name be honored as holy. Your kingdom come. Your will be done on earth as it is in heaven. Give us today our daily bread. And forgive us our debts, as we also have forgiven our debtors. Do not bring us into temptation but deliver us from the evil one. For Yours is the kingdom and the power and the glory forever. Amen." The Lord is faithful to answer our prayers. I **prayed** to the LORD, and he answered me. He freed me from all my fears. (Psalm 34:4, NLT).

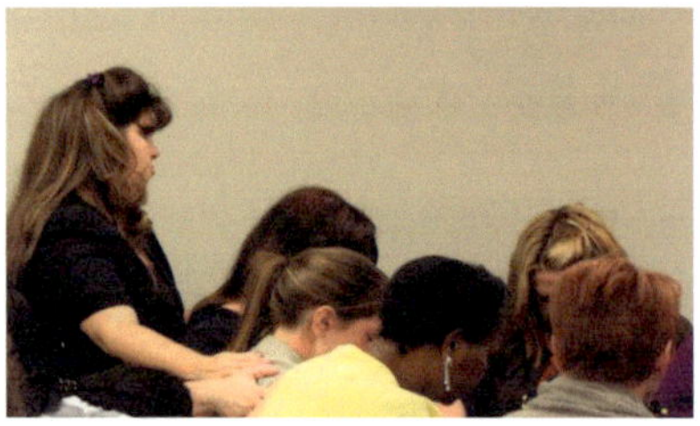

God is the author of life and deserves our praise. But each day the LORD pours his unfailing love upon me, and through each night I sing his songs, **praying** to God who gives me life (Psalm 42:8, NLT). I thank you for answering my **prayer** and giving me victory! (Psalm 118:21, NLT). As Doulas, we are called to be co-laborers with women and in the harvest field with Christ in our communities. He said to his disciples, "The harvest is great, but the workers are few. So, pray to the Lord who oversees the harvest; ask him to send more workers into his fields." (Matthew 9:37-38, NLT).

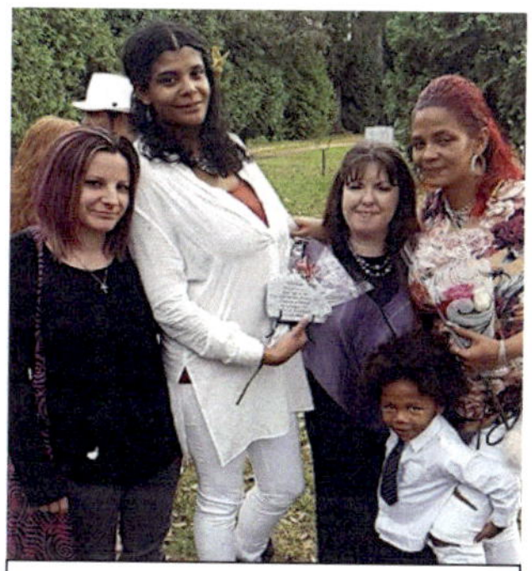

Erin, Morgan, Jessica and Jade have shared in the victories and the sorrows of life.

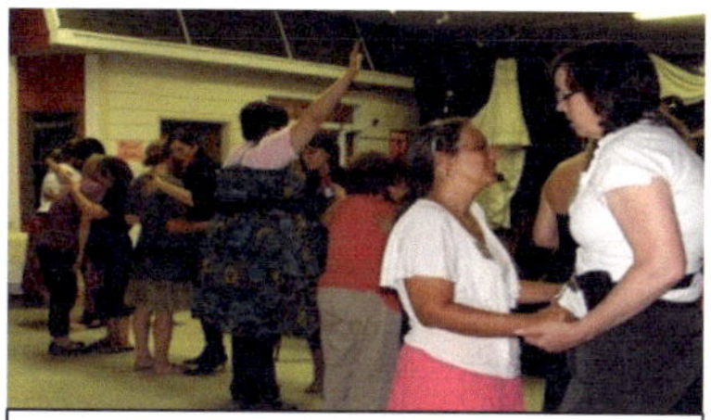

A tender moment was shared between Deb Teske, praying for Carol Boettcher at the first WOS conference (2011).

But when you are **praying**, first forgive anyone you are holding a grudge against, so that your Father in heaven will forgive your sins, too." (Mark 11:25, NLT). In the various circumstances, we find ourselves, whether physical or spiritual we need to remember to pray. James 5:13-15 says, "Are any of you suffering hardships? You should **pray**. Are any of you happy? You should sing praises. Are any of you sick? You should call for the elders of the church to come and **pray** over you, anointing you with oil in the name of the Lord. Such a **prayer** offered in faith will heal the sick, and the Lord will make you well. And if you have committed any sins, you will be forgiven."

Finally, Jude 1:20 admonishes us by saying, "You dear friends, must build each other up in your most holy faith, **pray** in the power of the Holy Spirit." In conclusion, we can come into agreement with this **prayer** from Ephesians 1:17-20 ... *"I **pray** for you constantly, asking God, the glorious Father of our Lord Jesus Christ, to give you spiritual wisdom and insight so that you might grow in your knowledge of God. I pray that your hearts will be flooded with light so that you can understand the confident hope He has given to those He called—his holy people who are His rich and glorious inheritance. I also **pray** that you will understand the incredible greatness of God's power for us who believe in him. This is the same mighty power that raised Christ from the dead and seated him in the place of honor at God's right hand in the heavenly realms."*

c.) **Discipleship**

“Jesus said to the people who believed in him, “You are truly my disciples if you remain faithful to my teachings. And you will know the truth, and the truth will set you free.” ...
“I have been given all authority in heaven and on earth. Therefore, go and make disciples of all the nations, baptizing them in the name of the Father and the Son and the Holy Spirit. Teach these new disciples to obey all the commands I have given you. And be sure of this: I am with you always, even to the end of the age.” (John 8:31-32; Matthew 28:18-20, NLT) ...

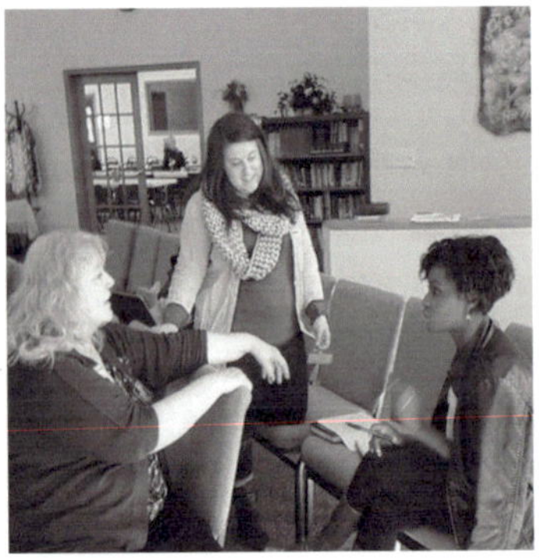

Left: Judi Heller, Samantha Carter, and Larissa Gronseth are engaged in the discipleship process through the ministry of the Women of Strength (2016).

Below: Rose Pixley, Deb Teske, Judi Heller, Stephanie Marsland, Lois Hancock, Jill Eidem, Julie Van Hook, and Jessica LaFavor show the importance of having spiritual mothers and discipleship.

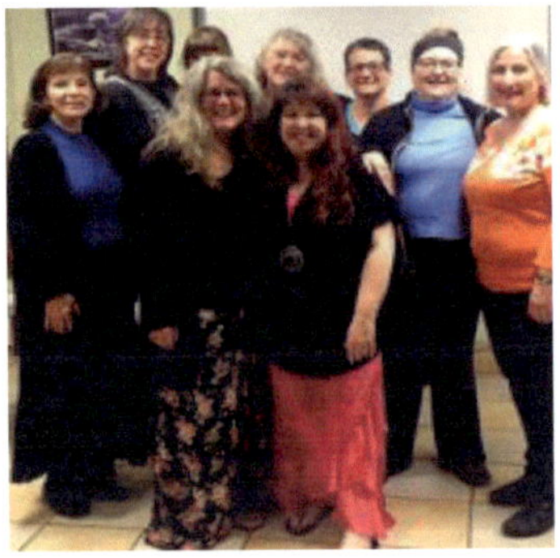

A disciple is a person who is a follower of a teacher, and they learn what they teach, by word, by action, and by example. A true disciple is a person who looks, acts, and speaks just like their teacher. Jesus is the truth; therefore, we need His Spirit to come into us and bring new life. This releases us to be who we are. In *Making Disciples* (2011), a children’s ministry curriculum, author Joanna Pixley wrote the following declaration to help train the next generation in discipleship. Discipleship has no age limitation; we must have a child-like faith if we are to inherit the Kingdom of God.

Discipleship Creed:

I will honor what’s right.

I will live by truth.

I will submit to authority.

I will shun evil.

And I will pray daily.

In John 13:34-35 Jesus tells us, “So now I am giving you a new commandment: Love each other. Just as I have loved you, you should love each other. Your love for one another will prove to the world that you are my disciples.” To be a disciple of Christ is to be a leader. In Matthew 20:26 Jesus said, “Whoever wants to be a leader among you must be your servant.” As Grateful Life Doulas, we are co-laborers of Christ and our communities; we know that our primary calling is to walk out the journey of new life with others.

CHAPTER 14

SPIRITUAL MENTORSHIP

DOULA DISCIPLESHIP

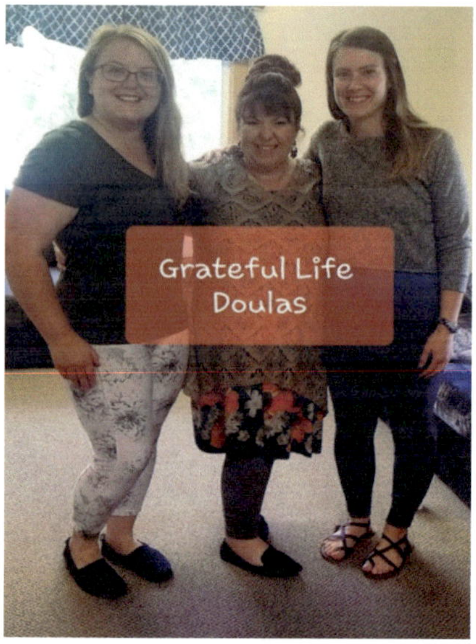

Left: Doula discipleship training—Sara, Jessica, and Anna.

Right: Katie and Justin Hawley right before the birth of their son, Judah.

Servant Leaders

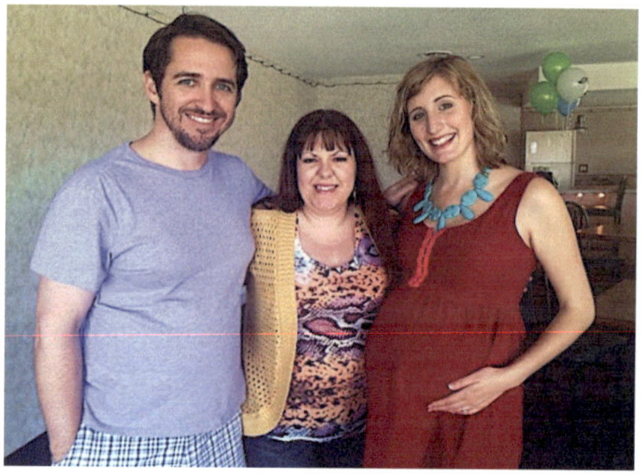

Doulos—Used approximately 160 in the New Testament.

*For you were called to freedom, brothers. Only do not use your freedom as an opportunity for the flesh but through love **serve** one another.* (Galatians 5:13).

Slave of Christ—1 Corinthians 7:22 and Titus 2:9-10 says, "Remember, if you were a slave when the Lord called you, then you are now free in the Lord. If you were free when the Lord called you, you are now a slave of Christ … Slaves must obey their masters and do their best to please them. They must not talk back or steal but must show themselves to be trustworthy and good. Then they will make the teaching about God our Savior attractive in every way." (NLT).

In God's Service—1 Corinthians 3:9 tells us, "For we are co-workers in God's service; you are God's field, God's building." Servanthood—Doulos is being a servant leader.

For the Kingdom of God—Colossians 4:11 reminds us of what we are doing here …
"They are working with me here for the kingdom of God … let us be grateful for a kingdom that cannot be shaken" (Hebrews 12:28).

Serve:

—Give oneself completely

—To the service of another

—Love in action everyday

—Honor others above yourself

—Have a heart of willingness

—No expectation of a reward

Qualities of a Servant of the Lord 2 Timothy 2:24 • Must not be quarrelsome • Must be kind to everyone • Able to teach • Not resentful

If we choose not to serve God, we will be a slave of something else …

- **Sin—**Slave to Sin Nature (John 8:34; Romans 6:17- 21; 2 Peter 2:19)
- **Fear—**Slave of Men (1 Corinthians 7:23) Slave to Fear (Romans 8:15; Hebrews 2:15)
- **Bondage—**Slave to Legalism (Galatians 4:8-9; 5:1) Slave to Money (Matthew 6:24)

"… **as for me and my house, we will serve the LORD**" (Joshua 24:15, NASB).

Deuteronomy 6:5—"You shall love the Lord your God with all your heart, with all your soul, and with all your strength" (NKJV).

Relationship Builders and Characteristics of a Leader:

<u>Trust, Responsibility, Confidence, Humility, Honesty, and Respect</u>

- Honor—treating everyone with dignity
- Empathy—putting yourself in someone else's shoes
- Awareness—knowing what is needed for yourself and others
- Persuasion—using your influence for good
- Vision—seeing the long-term goal
- Stewardship—to use your time, talents, and treasure well
- Commitment to the growth of others—empowerment
- Healing—ministry of Reconciliation
- Building community—outreach and loving our neighbor

Spiritual Mentoring:	**Discipleship Training:**
• Wedding/Marriage Materials	Bible Study/Prayer
• Children and Parenting	Deliverance/Identity
• Life Skills/Communication	Spiritual Recovery
• Purity Issues/Inner Healing	Apologetic/Worldview Resources

Admonition from the Word: Do Titus 2

Titus 2:3-5, 12-14 says, … "Teach women to live in a way that honors God. They must not slander others or be heavy drinkers. Instead, they should teach others what is good. These older women must train the younger women to love their husbands and their children, to live wisely and be pure, to work in their homes, to do good, and to be submissive to their husbands. Then they will not bring shame on the word of God … and we are instructed to turn from godless living and sinful pleasures. We should live in this evil world with wisdom, righteousness, and devotion to God as we look forward with hope to that wonderful day when the glory of our great God and Savior, Jesus Christ, will be revealed. He gave his life to free us from every kind of sin, to cleanse us, and to make us his very own people, committed to doing good deeds."

Ministry outline taken from Hebrews 13

- Let love continue, show hospitality, share what you have. (v. 1, 2, 16).
  (Fellowship meals, Bible study and Prayer).
- Remember those who are in prison and being mistreated. (v.3).
  (eg. *Next Chapter Ministries/ Voice of the Martyrs*).
- Let marriage be held in honor by all- having a biblical perspective. (v.4).
  (Pre-marital counseling, past purity issues, and current encouragement).
- Contentment, keeping your life free from the love of money. (v.5).
  (Budgeting, debt resources, financial freedom tools).
- Do not be led away by strange and diverse teachings. (v.9).
  (Apologetic studies and biblical worldview trainings).
- Let us continually offer up praise to God. (v.15).
  (Names of God, identity in Christ, expressions of praise and worship).

CARE: Mentor Model

<u>**C**ommitment, **A**ccountability, **R**espect, **E**xcellence</u>

Commitment is foundational for an atmosphere of trust to be built. Ministry doulas need to have a personal commitment to God. They must also have a commitment to the people they are mentoring.

Accountability is essential for continuing leadership training and support. Mentors or ministry doulas can be a part of the Grateful Life Doula Collective. This group will serve advisory purposes as well as ongoing spiritual equipping and prayer partnerships.

One must know how to show **Respect** to others when being a mentor. We want to show honor to all people as unique individuals created and valued by God. We do this by keeping our appointments and the information we are entrusted with confidential. Giving others the chance to share in a safe environment while we listen is a gift. Being respectful to our team members is another component of our integrity. When we communicate and treat those we are serving with respect, then we are being good examples as mentors.

A ministry of **Excellence** is what we strive for. Our heart is to shine the light of truth on a dark and dying world. When we allow the love of the Spirit to flow from us to others, it creates a place of hope and healing in our midst. Excellence in evangelism and knowing how to effectively share the gospel is a high priority. We are called to speak the truth in love to those we mentor. When we have a standard of excellence, it promotes security and trust.

To **CARE** means to minister to the spiritual needs of a person and to continue the work of discipleship. We have a fellowship of those who are diverse, yet like-minded in their desire to be co-laborers with Christ and their community. As ambassadors, we have been given a ministry of reconciliation for those who are lost, to declare the peace between God and man and to restore broken relationships.

EMBRACING MOMENTS HEALING JOURNAL

1.) From Our Heart to Yours

This is meant to be a time to share the gift of our life with other women after spending time alone in meditation. To contribute to their growth and healing through the strength of transparency. Write down a portion of your testimony and write a prayer of thanksgiving.

a. Your own testimony—share your story

b. A prayer from you—respond to the Lord

2.) A Word of Comfort

It may be different for everyone, but the Lord speaks to us so that we may have intimacy and grow in our faith. It is very important to take time to listen and feel His Spirit.

a. The love of God speaking—listen and write down or draw a picture

b. A Scripture Verse—look up a Bible passage

Reflection

Sometimes in dark places of our past or moments when we feel all alone, we need the reality and power of God's presence. When we know the truth of Christ, then it will set us free! Transformation happens through the renewing of our minds, will, and emotions; this is the restoration of our souls.

a. Ask Jesus the light to come and reveal the truth—record what is shown

b. Release your pain, receive healing from the Spirit—experience God

3.) Further Insights

This is a time to talk about how God has met you and what you have learned.
It is important that each woman knows she is in a safe place to share. Allow the co-laboring of ministry doulas to commence. After all the women share, have everyone write encouraging notes to the other women in the group. End in prayer

a. What did the Lord speak, show, and reveal to you? Group into pairs.

b. Where can wisdom be shared with another? This is doula discipleship …

CHAPTER 15

WOMEN OF STRENGTH

VIRTUES OF A WOMAN OF STRENGTH

1.) **Co-laborer**: One who partners with the work of Christ for His purposes. Being a co-laborer requires being a **servant** and **compassion**.

Two are better than one ... we are God's fellow workers; you are God's field and *building.* Ecclesiastes 4:9, 1 Corinthians 3:9

a.) **Servant:** Philippians 2:4-7

Have this mind among yourselves, which is yours in Christ Jesus, who, though he was in the form of God, did not count equality with God a thing to be grasped, but emptied himself, by taking the form of a servant, being born in the likeness of men.

b.) **Compassion:** Colossians 3:12-14

Put on then, as God's chosen ones … compassionate hearts, kindness, humility, meekness, and patience, bearing with one another and, if one has a complaint against another, forgiving each other; as the Lord has forgiven you, so you also must forgive… Above all this put-on love, which binds everything together in perfect harmony.

2.) **Hospitality:** The art of welcoming or inviting someone to have a place of belonging. Making time for relationship...when a woman is coming into spiritual new life, she needs to have a safe place to be. Your **attitude** and **preparation** are essential in helping her to feel embraced throughout this journey.

a.) **Attitude:** 1 Peter 4:8-11, Philippians 2:3—"Do nothing from selfish ambition or conceit, but in humility count others more significant than yourselves."

b.) **Preparation:** Proverbs 31:10-31, Be a woman of noble character.

3.) **Communication:** *Let your speech always be with grace, seasoned with salt, that you may know how you ought to answer each one.* (Colossians 4:6).

We need to be able to communicate verbally, physically, and emotionally. Being able to understand and relay pertinent information is important when we minister to others. As servants, we must be able to **listen** intently as well as **understand** a language not necessarily spoken with words. Effective communication with women is an essential skill whether we are coaching in mentorship, doing inner healing prayer or teaching.

a.) **Listening**—1 Peter 3:4

You should clothe yourselves instead with the beauty that comes from within, the unfading beauty of a gentle and quiet spirit, which is so precious to God.

This will enable us to hear God's still small voice in any circumstance that we may face.

b.) **Understanding—**Colossians 1:9-14

As we are filled with the knowledge of God's will, spiritual wisdom and understanding become ours. This is so that we may be empowered through the Holy Spirit to do the work God has called us to as His servants.

Luke 10:39—She had a sister called Mary, who was seated at the Lord's feet, listening to His word. We like Mary must learn to listen to those we are mistering to. As ministry doulas, it is important to recognize our role as we participate in the process of walking alongside those on the journey of new life. It is an honor to be a part of such an intimate moment with others. We must remember to reflect the heart Jesus as we continue the work we have been called to. Having a grateful life comes from knowing the love of Christ and partnering with Him to touch others with that same love as well.

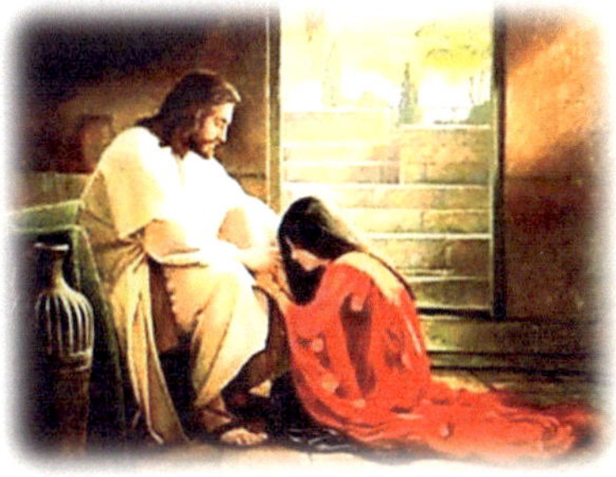

Poem: A Strong Woman vs. A Woman of Strength

A strong woman works out every day to keep her body in shape, but a woman of strength kneels in prayer to keep her soul in shape ...

A strong woman isn't afraid of anything, but a woman of strength shows courage in the midst of her fear ...

A strong woman won't let anyone get the best of her, but a woman of strength gives the best of her to everyone ...

A strong woman makes mistakes and avoids the same in the future, but a woman of strength realizes life's mistakes can also be God's blessings and capitalizes on them ...

A strong woman walks sure footedly, but a woman of strength knows God will catch her when she falls …

A strong woman wears the look of confidence on her face, but a woman of strength wears grace ...

A strong woman has faith that she is strong enough for the journey, but a woman of strength has faith that it is in the journey that she will become strong ...

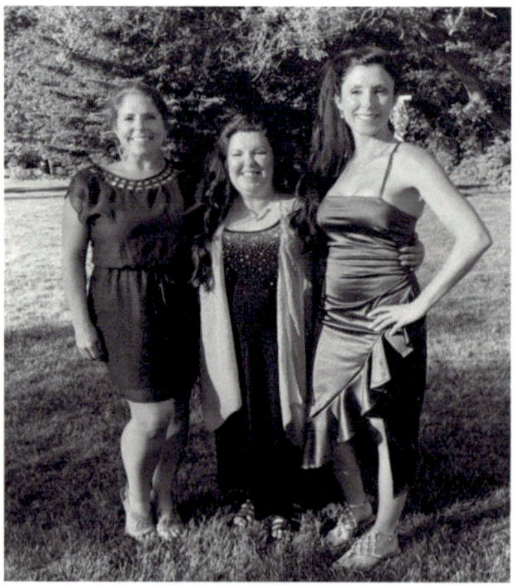

Me and my two sisters, Jennifer, and Joanna

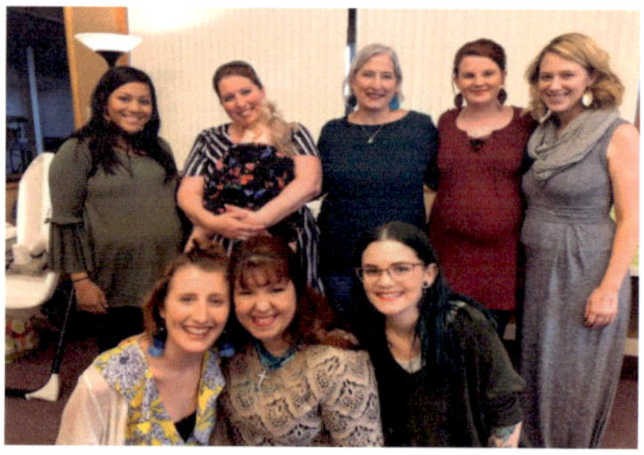

Sarita, Amanda, Jill, Jamie, and Hannah- top. Katie, Jessica, and Eden- below. These sisters in Christ share more than birth and motherhood…they have stories to tell and strength to give.

TREASURES OF THE HEART

Mary, the mother of Jesus, a true woman of strength

1. There was a **sign**—pregnancy and birth
2. There was a **seed**—the word spoken
3. There was a **season**—promise fulfilled

Isaiah 7:14— "All right then, the Lord himself will give you the sign.
Look! The virgin will conceive a child! She will give birth to a son and will call him Immanuel (which means 'God is with us')."

1. There was a **sign**—pregnancy of Mary and the birth of Jesus

Matthew 1:18- 23. This is how the birth of Jesus the Messiah came about: His mother Mary was pledged to be married to Joseph, but before they came together, she was found to be pregnant through the Holy Spirit. Because Joseph her husband was faithful to the law, and yet did not want to expose her to public disgrace, he had in mind to divorce her quietly. But after he had considered this, an angel of the Lord appeared to him in a dream and said, "Joseph son of David, do not be afraid to take Mary home as your wife, because what is conceived in her is from the Holy Spirit. She will give birth to a son, and you are to give him the name Jesus because he will save his people from their sins." All this took place to fulfill what the Lord had said through the prophet: "The virgin will conceive and give birth to a son, and they will call him Immanuel."

Luke 24 Joseph also went up from the town of Nazareth in Galilee to Judea, to Bethlehem the town of David (Beloved), because he belonged to the house and line of David. He went there to register with Mary, who was pledged to be married to him and was expecting a child. While they were there, the time came for the baby to be born, and she gave birth to her firstborn, a son. She wrapped him in cloths and placed him in a manger because there was no guest room available for them. And there were shepherds living out in the fields nearby, keeping watch over their flocks at night. An angel of the Lord appeared to them, and the glory of the Lord shone around them, and they were terrified. But the angel said to them, "Do not be afraid. I bring you **good news** that will cause great joy for all the people. Today in the town of David a Savior has been born to you; he is the Messiah, the Lord. This will be a **sign** to you: You will find a baby wrapped in cloths and lying in a manger."

Why was Jesus laying in a manger in swaddling clothes a sign to these shepherds?

Micah 4:8 gives some insight, *"As for you, O watchtower of the flock [Hebrew Migdal Eder], O stronghold of the daughter of Zion, the former dominion will be restored to you; kingship will come to the Daughter of Jerusalem."* Migdal Eder was a watchtower located in the northern part of Bethlehem built to protect the Temple flocks. [1]"During the lambing season the sheep were brought there from the fields, as the lower level was the birthing room for sacrificial lambs." [2] Priestly shepherds "would wrap the newborn lambs in swaddling clothes" and place them in a manger "until they calmed down" [3] to keep them "without defect" [4]suitable to be sacrificial lambs for the sin of the Israelites. Bethlehem was special because the shepherds in the fields of Bethlehem raised lambs for the Jewish temple in Jerusalem. The shepherds who heard the angels and came to see the baby Jesus knew the significance of the birth of a sacrificial lamb, and this is what Jesus became. The angels did not have to tell the shepherds precisely where to go in Bethlehem to find Jesus, because there was only one place where sacrificial lambs were birthed, the cave under the watch tower of Migdal Edar.

1 Alfred Edersheim, The life and times of Jesus the Messiah, book 2, pg 131

2 Charles E. McCracken, For you and me, Israel My Glory, Nov/Dec 2008 pg 25.

3 Jimmy DeYoung, "Jimmy's Prophetic Perspective on the News," Dec 23, 2005.

4 Leviticus 4:32

5 Abrams, C. P. Where was the birthplace of the Lord Jesus? **http://www.bibletruth.org/BirthPlaceofJesus.html**

Why did God choose to reveal the incarnation to humble shepherds in the first place?

Jesus was born in Bethlehem, the city of David. Messiah would come through the lineage of David, who was a shepherd before he became a king. Jesus was born a king but revealed Himself first as a shepherd in John 10:22-28. *It was now winter, and Jesus was in Jerusalem at the time of Hanukkah, the Festival of Dedication or of Lights. He was in the Temple, walking through the section known as Solomon's Colonnade. The people surrounded him and asked, "How long are you going to keep us in suspense? If you are the Messiah, tell us plainly." Jesus replied, "I have already told you, and you don't believe me. The proof is the work I do in my father's name. But you don't believe me because you are not my sheep. My sheep listen to my voice; I know them, and they follow me. I give them eternal life, and they will never perish. No one can snatch them away from me …* Ezekiel 34 is a traditional passage that is read at

Hanukkah—listen to these words, [11] *For thus says the Lord GOD, "Behold, I Myself will search for My sheep and seek them out ...* [15a] *I will feed My flock and I will lead them to rest," declares the Lord GOD.* [16] *"I will seek the lost, bring back the scattered, bind up the broken and strengthen the sick ...* [23b] *"Then I will set over them one shepherd, my servant David, and he will feed them; he will feed them himself and be their shepherd ...*

Isn't it interesting that at the celebration for the rededication of the temple and festival of lights the light of the world, Jesus reveals Himself as Messiah! Worship is going from inside the temple to inside of you and me, we are now the temple of God, where He dwells. Some were waiting for this fulfillment to come to pass!

2. There was a **seed**—the **word** spoken by the Lord, prophets, and others who marveled. (Greek word is **sperma**, meaning the source of all life).

Let's go back to Luke chapter 2 … "When the angels had left them and gone into heaven, the shepherds said to one another, 'Let's go to Bethlehem and see this thing that has happened, which the Lord has told us about.' So, they hurried off and found Mary and Joseph, and the baby, who was lying in the manger. When they had seen him, **they spread the word** concerning what had been told them about this child, and all who heard it were amazed at what the shepherds said to them. **Mary treasured up all these things and pondered them in her heart.** The shepherds returned, glorifying and praising God for all the things they had heard and seen, which were just as they had been told. On the eighth day, when it was time to circumcise the child, he was named Jesus, the name the angel had given him before he was conceived … Now there was a man in Jerusalem called Simeon, who was righteous and devout. He was waiting for the consolation of Israel, and the Holy Spirit was on him. It had been revealed to him by the Holy Spirit that he would not die before he had seen the Lord's Messiah. Moved by the Spirit, he went into the temple courts. When the parents brought in the child Jesus to do for him what the custom of the Law required, Simeon took him in his arms and praised God, saying: 'Sovereign Lord, as you have promised, you may now dismiss your servant in peace.

For my eyes have seen your salvation, which you have prepared in the sight of all nations: a **light for revelation** to the Gentiles, and the glory of your people Israel.' The child's father and mother marveled at what was said about him. Then Simeon blessed them and said to Mary, his mother: 'This child is destined to cause the falling and rising of many in Israel, and to be a sign that will be spoken against, so that the thoughts of many hearts will be revealed. And a sword will pierce your own soul too' … And the child grew and became strong; he was filled with wisdom, and the grace of God was on him."

Whether the fruit of the ground or the fruit of womb, all life begins with a seed. The parable of the sower, Matthew 13:44-46, tells us that God's Word is like a seed planted, ready to produce a harvest (spiritual new life)! In the parable of the "Hidden Treasure and Pearl of Great Price," the Bible tells us that: "The kingdom of heaven is like treasure hidden in a field." When a man found it, he hid it again, and then in his joy went and sold all he had and bought that field. Seeds are planted in the ground, but the Gospel is planted in our hearts. We spread the gospel like scattering seeds.

"Again, the kingdom of heaven is like a merchant looking for fine pearls. When he found one of great value, he went away and sold everything he had and bought it. May we do as Psalm 119:11 says, "Your word have I treasured [hidden] in my heart, that I may not sin against you." Mary hid the treasure of truth, all the words spoken about Jesus! Jesus is the source of all life- John 1:1-4 says, "In the beginning was the Word, and the Word was with God, and the Word was God. He was with God in the beginning. Through him all things were made; without him nothing was made that has been made. In him was life, and that life was the light of all mankind."

3. There was a **season**—promise fulfilled.

Isaiah 43:19—"See, I am doing a new thing! Now it springs up; do you not perceive it? I am making a way in the wilderness and streams in the wasteland." What springs up first must be planted-God's promises will come to fruition! The impact that the truth of the Word makes in a person is the same as it was in Jesus' day-Matthew 4:23,24 says, "*Proclaiming the gospel of the kingdom, He went about healing every disease and every affliction among the people … they brought him all the sick, those afflicted with various diseases and pains, those oppressed by demons, epileptics, and paralytics, and Jesus healed them*." This is what the Prophet Isaiah foretold: Isaiah 42:6-7, 58:6-12, *"I am the LORD; I have called you in righteousness; I will take you by the hand and keep you; I will give you as a covenant for the people, a light for the nations, to open the eyes that are blind, to bring out the prisoners from the dungeon, from the prison those who sit in darkness …"*

"This is the kind of fasting I want: Free those who are wrongly imprisoned; lighten the burden of those who work for you. Let the oppressed go free and remove the chains that bind people.[7] Share your food with the hungry and give shelter to the homeless. Give clothes to those who need them, and do not hide from relatives who need your help. "Then your salvation will come like the dawn and your wounds will quickly heal. Your godliness will lead you forward, and the glory of the LORD will protect you from behind. Then when you call, the LORD will answer. 'Yes, I am here,' he will quickly reply. "Remove the heavy yoke of oppression. Stop pointing your finger and spreading vicious rumors! Feed the hungry and help those in trouble. Then your light will shine out from the darkness, and the darkness around you will be as bright as noon. The LORD will guide you continually, giving you water when you are dry and restoring your strength. You will be like a well-watered garden, like an ever-flowing spring. Some of you will rebuild the deserted ruins of your cities. Then you will be known as a rebuilder of walls and a restorer of homes." Our promises are already here in the spirit, we are just waiting for the manifestation to appear. Until then, we like Mary will treasure all these things in our hearts.

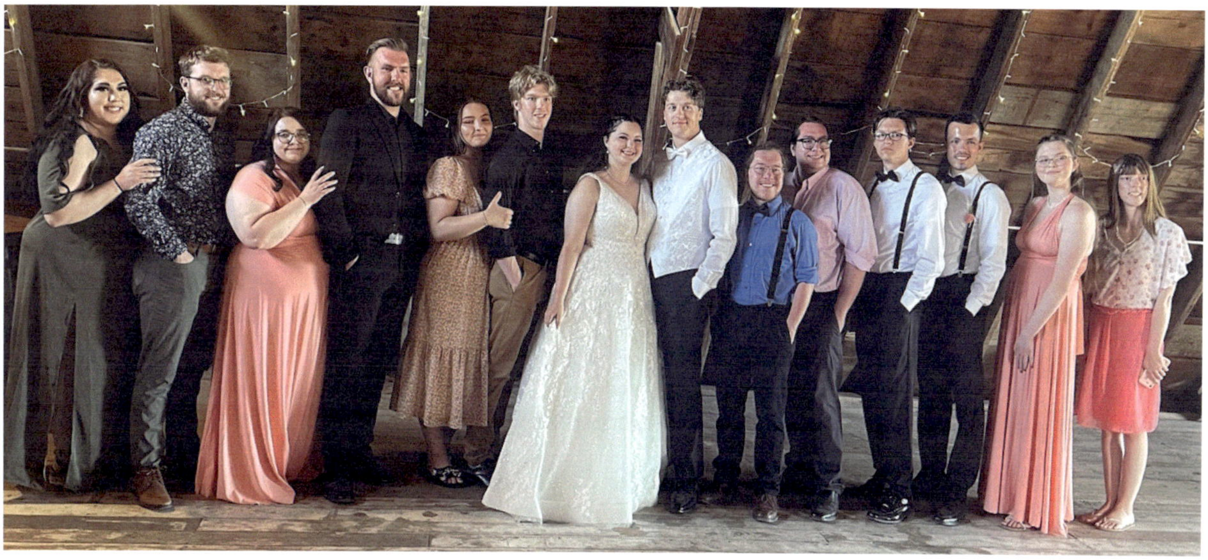

Maricella, Colin, Abby, Samuel, Jess, Noah, Faith, Isaac, Alejandro, Antonio, David, Isaiah, Olivia, and Christine are the treasures of my heart! They represent generational blessings, freedom, and new beginnings. As a mother, a doula for both of my sisters and an Auntie, I learned how to shepherd my family before walking the path of ministry.

WOMEN IN MINISTRY

God created men and women in His image to govern and reign over creation together.

Genesis 1:27- "So God created human beings in his own image. In the image of God, He created them; male and female he created them. [28] Then God blessed them and said, 'Be fruitful and multiply. Fill the earth and govern it. Reign over the fish in the sea, the birds in the sky, and all the animals that scurry along the ground.'"

Women Prophets: Miriam, Deborah, Huldah, Isaiah's wife, Anna, Daughters of Phillip.

Exodus 15:20—hen **Miriam the prophet**, Aaron's sister, took a tambourine and led the women as they played their tambourines and danced. 21 And Miriam sang this song: "Sing to the LORD, for he has triumphed gloriously; he has hurled both horse and rider into the sea." Judges 4:4—Now **Deborah, a prophetess**, the wife of Lappidoth, **was judging Israel**. Besides being a prophetess, Deborah was a judge. As told in the book of Judges, Deborah is the fourth judge to lead the nation of Israel (Judges 4:1-5:31). The Hebrew word for judge is "shaphat" which means "to deliver" or "to rule."

Kings 22:14—So Hilkiah the priest, Ahikam, Achbor, Shaphan, and Asaiah went to **Huldah the prophetess**, the wife of Shallum the son of Tikvah, the son of Harhas, keeper of the wardrobe.
(She dwelt in Jerusalem in the Second Quarter.) And they spoke with her.
Huldah is a prophetess mentioned in 2 Kings 22:14-20 and 2 Chronicles 34:22-28. She was a contemporary of the prophet Jeremiah, during the reign of King Josiah.

The major prophet **Isaiah considered his wife to be a prophetess**
Isaiah 8:3—"And I went unto the prophetess; and she conceived and bare a son.
Then said the LORD to me, Call his name Mahershalalhashbaz.

Anna is a prophetess that bears witness to the redeemer. She is mentioned in Luke 2:36-38. She was very old and spent all her time worshiping God by fasting and praying at the temple. Upon seeing the baby Jesus, she praised God; she joyfully told of the child to everyone in the community seeking deliverance for Jerusalem.

Acts 21:8-9—On the next day we who were Paul's companions departed and came to Caesarea, and entered the house of Philip the evangelist, who was one of the seven, and stayed with him. Now **this man had four virgin daughters who prophesied.**

The Greek word used in Acts 21:9 for prophesying is prophēteuō, "*to prophesy, to be a prophet, speak forth by divine inspirations, to predict.*" The gift of prophesy operating on Phillip's daughters is the fulfillment of another prophesy. The prophet Joel foretold in Joel 2:28 that when the Holy Spirit would be poured out "your sons and daughters shall prophesy." Acts 2:17 reaffirms Joel's Old Testament prophesy.

Other women leaders:

Lydia – businesswoman who became a central leader in the Philippian Church
Priscilla – helped Paul establish churches at Corinth and Ephesus; corrected Apollo's preaching
Junias – an Apostle
Phoebe – deacon; commended by Paul for her service to the church.

Being a servant of the Lord:

Proverbs 31:26- She opens her mouth with wisdom, and the teaching of kindness is on her tongue. 1 Timothy 1:5- I am reminded of your sincere faith, a faith that dwelt first in your grandmother Lois and your mother Eunice and now, I am sure, dwells in you as well. 2 Timothy 2:15, 24, 25—"Do your best to present yourself to God as one approved, a worker who has no need to be ashamed, rightly handling the word of truth ... and the Lord's servant must not be quarrelsome but kind to everyone, able to teach, patiently enduring evil, correcting opponents with gentleness." God may perhaps grant them repentance leading to a knowledge of the truth...

Jesus did have a number of women among His larger circle of disciples.
(Matthew 27:55-56, Mark 15:40-41, Luke 8:1-3, 23:49, John 20:14-18).
Several women held important positions in the early Christian churches.
Acts 1:14—They all met together and were constantly united in prayer, along with Mary the mother of Jesus, several other women, and the brothers of Jesus. (18:24-26, 21:7-9, Romans 16:1-16).

Although he accepted that people may have different roles in society, the apostle **Paul proclaimed that all believers are equal in God's sight**: "You are all sons of God through faith in Christ Jesus, for all of you who were baptized into Christ have clothed yourselves with Christ.

There is neither Jew nor Greek, slave nor free, male nor female, **for you are all one in Christ Jesus.** If you belong to Christ, then you are Abraham's seed, and heirs according to the promise." (NIV, Galatians 3:26-29)

Ephesians 4:11-13, "And he gave some, apostles; and some, prophets; and some, evangelists; and some, pastors and teachers; For the perfecting of the saints, for the work of the ministry, for the edifying of the body of Christ: Till we all come in the unity of the faith, and of the knowledge of the Son of God, unto a perfect man, unto the measure of the stature of the fullness of Christ: …"

The first evangelists were women:

"Early on Sunday morning, as the new day was dawning, Mary Magdalene and the other Mary went out to visit the tomb ... Then the angel spoke to the women. 'Don't be afraid!' he said. 'I know you are looking for Jesus, who was crucified. He isn't here! He is risen from the dead, just as he said would happen. Come, see where his body was lying. And now, go quickly and tell his disciples that he has risen from the dead, and he is going ahead of you to Galilee. You will see him there. Remember what I have told you.' The women ran quickly from the tomb. They were very frightened but also filled with great joy, and they rushed to give the disciples the angel's message. And as they went, Jesus met them and greeted them. And they ran to him, grasped his feet, and worshiped him. Then Jesus said to them, 'Don't be afraid! Go tell my brothers to leave for Galilee, and they will see me there'" (Matthew 28:1, 5-10).

Luke 24:9—"So they rushed back from the tomb to tell his eleven disciples—and everyone else—what had happened. [10]It was Mary Magdalene, Joanna, Mary the mother of James, and several other women who told the apostles what had happened."

The first thing God ever told His children to do was to "Be fruitful and multiply" (Genesis 1:28). The last thing Jesus ever said to His disciples was to "Go into all the world and preach the gospel to everyone…and make disciples of all nations" (Mark 16:15, Matthew 28:19). He gave us a heart for new life and legacy!

CONCLUSION

"The concept of having a companion providing support to women is an ancient practice, evidenced by archeological findings of stone carvings and statues and anthropological studies. However, the contemporary role of "doula" first emerged from the natural birth movement in the US in the 1960s when women began desiring unmedicated, low-intervention births and began to have friends and others with formal or practical knowledge about childbirth provide them with support during pregnancy. Women came back to sharing the spiritual wisdom that had always been theirs. This important shift brought birth back to a place of social celebration.

Grateful Life is about becoming healthy, growing, and full of love in every area.

Why not start at the beginning?

One thing we focus on is spiritual mentorship for women in our communities and around the world! We want you to experience empowerment and encouragement that will change your life and equip you to walk in victory. We acknowledge the parallel of the spiritual and physical new life, so we also provide Christ-centered childbirth education and doula training. At no other time in history has it been so crucial that women and families have the support necessary to choose life! As we provide the essential components of information and application to those who have the heart to serve women experiencing unplanned pregnancy, lives will be saved!

Our goal is to teach about pregnancy and motherhood from a spiritual perspective to cultivate a love at birth and love for life. When we show love for a mother at the birth of her baby, she is empowered and can continue to invest in herself, which will allow her love to flow to her child as well. We also mentor women in the art of becoming professional doulas so that they can assist birthing mothers with confidence and compassion.

Thank you for being a part of the solution and growing yourself in ways that will impact the world around you. Every mother who feels supported, unafraid and knows that she's not alone will be empowered through this journey of new life to love herself and her baby.

We as co-laborers provide presence and peace for her to find the truth she was born with.

This is where change starts, one life at a time! May you always have the heart of a doula and birth your own vision.

APPENDICES

Code of Ethics: Birth Doula* DONA International (2017)

I. Rules of Conduct

A. Propriety.

The doula should maintain high standards of personal conduct… as a birth doula.

B. Competence and Professional Development.

The doula should strive to become and remain proficient in the professional practice and the performance of professional functions through continuing education, affiliation with related organizations, and associations with other birth doulas.

C. Honor our Statement of Values on Social Media.

On social media platforms, the doula should extend respect, courtesy, fairness and good faith towards doulas and on behalf of the doula profession. The influence on students, consumers and fellow doulas extends beyond time in a birth, postpartum session or workshop setting. When engaging on social media platforms, the doula agrees to clarify that any opinions are his/her own, show respect in each communication, use good judgment in sharing only public information, and be aware that social media content is permanent…

D. Integrity.

The doula should act in accordance with the highest standards of professional integrity.

II. Ethical Responsibility to Clients

A. Primacy of Client's Interests.

The doula's primary responsibility is to his/her clients.

B. Rights and Prerogatives of Clients.

The doula should make every effort to foster maximum self-determination on the part of his/her clients.

C. Confidentiality and Privacy.

The doula should respect the privacy of clients and hold in confidence all information obtained in the course of professional service.

D. Obligation to Serve.

The doula should assist each client seeking birth doula support either by providing services or making appropriate referrals.

E. Reliability.

When the doula agrees to work with a particular client, his/her obligation is to do so reliably, without fail, for the term of the agreement.

F. Fees.

When setting fees, the doula should ensure that they are fair, reasonable, and commensurate with services performed. The doula must clearly state his/her fees to the client and describe the services provided, terms of payment and refund policies.

III. Ethical Responsibility to Colleagues

A. Respect, Fairness, and Courtesy.

The doula should treat colleagues with respect, courtesy, fairness, and good faith…we do not tolerate discrimination (including age, sex, race, color, creed, religion, ethnicity, sexual orientation, gender identity, national origin, citizenship, disability, or marital status or any other legally recognized protected group) and will uphold federal, state, and local laws, regulations or ordinances.

B. Dealing with Colleagues' Clients.

The doula has the responsibility to relate to the clients of colleagues with full professional consideration.

IV. Ethical Responsibility to the Birth Doula Profession

A. Maintaining the Integrity of the Profession.

The doula should uphold and advance the values, ethics, knowledge and mission of the profession. The doula is encouraged to promote the DONA International vision of "A doula for every person who wants one," by providing birth doula services at a reduced cost, if possible, or making appropriate referrals, as available.

V. Ethical Responsibility to Society

A. Promoting Maternal and Child Welfare.

The doula should promote the general health of women and their babies, and whenever possible, that of their family and friends as well.

Standards of Practice: Birth Doula

I. Scope

A. Services Rendered.

The doula accompanies the woman in labor, provides emotional and Physical support, suggests comfort measures, and provides support and suggestions for the partner. Whenever possible, the doula provides pre- and post-partum emotional support, including explanation and discussion of practices and procedures, and assistance in acquiring the knowledge necessary for the client to make informed decisions about their own care. Additionally, as doulas do not "prescribe" treatment, any suggestions or information provided within the role of the doula must be done with the provision that the doula advises his/her client to check with the primary care provider before using any application.

B. Limits to Practice.

DONA International Standards and Certification apply to emotional, physical and informational support only. The DONA certified or member doula does not perform clinical or medical tasks, such as taking blood pressure or temperature, fetal heart tone checks, vaginal examinations, or postpartum clinical care. They will not diagnose or treat in any modality.

i. If the doula has qualifications in alternative or complementary modalities (such as aromatherapy, childbirth education, massage therapy, placenta encapsulation, etc.), s/he must make it very clear to her/his clients and others that those modalities are an additional service, outside of the doula's scope of practice.

ii. A healthcare provider (such as a nurse, midwife, chiropractor, etc.) may not refer to her/himself as a doula while providing services outside of a doula's scope of practice.

C. Advocacy.

The doula advocates for the client's wishes as expressed in her birth plan, in prenatal conversations, and in intrapartum discussion, by encouraging his/her client to ask questions of her care provider and to express her preferences and concerns. Clients and doulas must recognize that the advocacy role does not include the doula speaking instead of the client or making decisions for the client …

D. Referrals.

For client needs beyond the scope of the doula's training, referrals are made to appropriate resources.

II. Continuity of Care

A. **The doula should make backup arrangements** with another doula to ensure services to the client if the doula is unable to attend the birth. Should any doula feel a need to discontinue service to an established client, it is the doula's responsibility to notify the client in writing and arrange for a replacement, if the client so desires. This may be accomplished by: Introducing the client to the backup doula. Following up with the client or backup doula to make sure the client's needs are being accommodated.

III. Training and Experience

A. **Training-** Completion of a DONA International-ap birth doula workshop is but one step in the process of training and certification. Doulas who are certified by DONA International will have completed all the requirements as set forth in the DONA International Requirements for Birth Doula Certification.

B. **Experience-** Doulas certified by DONA International will have the experience as set forth in the DONA International Requirements for Birth Doula Certification.

C. **Maintenance of Certification-** DONA doulas will maintain certification as outlined in the DONA recertification packet. Must be completed each three-year period of practice.

<table>
<tr><th colspan="3">Grateful Life Team Membership Application</th></tr>
<tr><td colspan="2">Name:</td><td>Phone:</td></tr>
<tr><td colspan="3">Experience:</td></tr>
<tr><td>Date of birth:</td><td colspan="2">Email:</td></tr>
<tr><td colspan="3">Tell us how you would like to use your time, talents, and treasures for Grateful Life Doula Collective. Please mark which positions you are interested in.</td></tr>
<tr><td colspan="3">Birth/ Postpartum Doula   On-call Child Care
Trauma Healing   Community Resource List
Mentorship   Prayer Team- Intercessory/ Prophetic</td></tr>
<tr><td>How Long would you like to serve?</td><td>12-18 months</td><td>18-36 months</td></tr>
<tr><td colspan="3">How would you describe your relationship with God?

Have you made a commitment to follow Jesus or been baptized by the Holy Spirit?</td></tr>
<tr><td colspan="3">References</td></tr>
<tr><td>Name</td><td>Email</td><td>Phone</td></tr>
<tr><td></td><td></td><td></td></tr>
<tr><td></td><td></td><td></td></tr>
<tr><td colspan="2">Signature of applicant:</td><td>Date:</td></tr>
<tr><td colspan="3">Disclaimer: We are not doing background checks currently. Membership payment due upon acceptance.</td></tr>
</table>

Description of Products and Services:

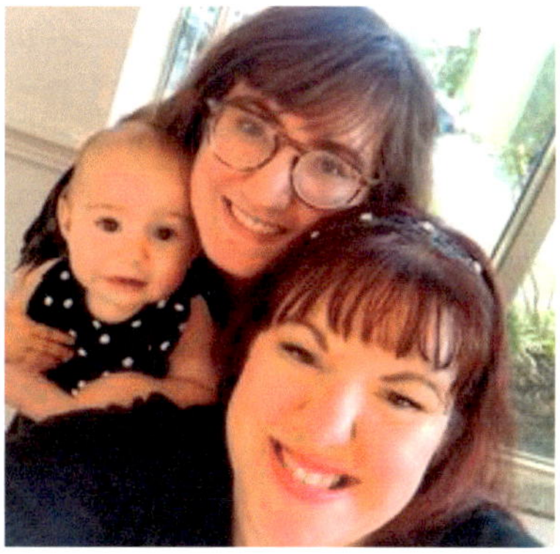

Families served

- Childbirth Education
- Birth Planning/ Consultation
- Trauma Healing for Mothers
- Labor and Delivery Support
- Newborn Care Plan/ Postpartum Services

Doulas

Christian Doula Training	Seminars 1.5-2hrs. classroom style
• Seminars	Training sessions for specific skills
• Workshop	2-day interactive workshop
• Manual	6–8-week classes
• Retreats	Weekends

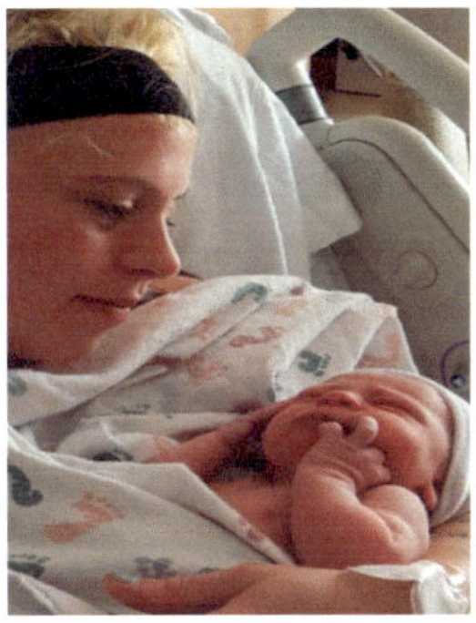

Birth: Consultation/3hrs. (Childbirth education only)

Birth Package: phone support, pre-natal meetings, labor, and aftercare

Postpartum: Breastfeeding support, listening, goal setting, light cleaning, cooking, sibling care, and trauma processing.

Prices vary for independent doulas.

Doulas	**Families**
Independent	Multigenerational
Doula teams	Faith declared or not
Families/Individuals	Various social economic status
Community resources	All ethnicities
Education	Group support

Birth Doula Agreement: What is my role as a birth doula?

As a Birth Doula, I accompany women in labor to help ensure a safe and satisfying birth experience. I have completed the doula training workshop through Grateful Life Ministries LLC. I draw on my professional training, knowledge, and experiences to provide physical, emotional, and information support to families. I can provide reassurance and perspective to you and your partner, make suggestions for labor progress, and help with relaxation, massage, positioning, and other techniques for comfort. I am independent and self-employed. As your doula, I am working for you, not your caregiver or the facility where you choose to give birth.

Consultation/Confidentiality

This initial meeting is free and does not obligate you to use my services. If you choose to select me as your doula, I will want to become more familiar with your plans for labor, birth, and postpartum. I do expect to meet at least twice before labor to become acquainted and to plan how we might best work together. I will keep our conversations and details about your care confidential unless there is a cause for concern. I ask for permission to write details and share information with the understanding that it is for those working directly with you and your family and it is for the benefit of your care as well as for data purposes. This contract will be signed at or before the first prenatal meeting.

Prenatal meetings

I prefer we arrange for 2 prenatal meetings (1-2 hours), preferably before 37 weeks in your pregnancy. This meeting gives us a chance to talk in detail about your preferences regarding your birth. If you have a Birth Plan, we will review it carefully. I will want to know how you and your partner foresee working together, and the roles of others who may be attending the birth. We can discuss together what fears and concerns you have regarding the birth. We can review your preferences regarding the use of pain medications. I will also inform you of times when I am unavailable for labor support. To cover those times, I will arrange one or more qualified back-up doulas whom you may also meet.

When Labor Begins

When you think labor has begun, call me so we can begin making arrangements for the birth. We will check in every few hours by phone. It is up to you to decide at what point in your labor you want me to come and be with you. Once you make that choice, I will generally be there within an hour, and will remain with you until after the birth.

During Labor

I can offer help and advice with comfort measures such as patterned breathing, focused relaxation, encouraging movement, suggesting positions for labor, and doing massage. I can assist with gathering information about the progress of labor to make sure you have the information you need to make informed decisions about your birth. I can also serve as an advocate when needed. I provide continuous emotional reassurance throughout labor and delivery, as well as spiritual support when requested.

After the Delivery

I expect to remain with a client for 1-2 hours after birth until you are comfortable, and the family is ready for quiet time together. I can also help with breastfeeding. My services include one postpartum visit, usually within two weeks of the birth. During this visit, I can provide breastfeeding support, baby care tips, referrals to community resources, and a chance to discuss the birth experience.

As a doula, I do not:

Perform clinical tasks, such as blood pressure, fetal heart checks, vaginal exams, etc. I am there to provide professional non-medical support. I will help you get the information necessary to make informed decisions. I will discuss your concerns with you and suggest options, but it is always best if you or your partner can speak directly to the clinical staff.

Contract

The total fee for my services is $__________. I am open to payment plans all fees are due by 37 weeks. Upon signing of this contract, a non-refundable deposit, in the amount of $250 or a third of the agreed-upon fee, is due. Once you sign the contract and the deposit is paid, your due date is officially scheduled on my calendar.

Fulfillment of Labor Support includes the following circumstances:

- Elective Cesarean
- C-section after trial of labor
- Rapid Labor
- Epidural or pain medication where family rest allows for doula to take a break
- Family does not contact doula at time of labor or unscheduled induction
- Any portion of services in which the client chooses not to take advantage of the full doula services herein agreed to. (i.e. does not schedule their postpartum visit, change of mind about birth support.)

Liability

Grateful Life Ministries LLC is covered by CM&F Group Inc. and will not be held liable for any damages, court-related costs or suits naming the doula. As a Grateful Life Doula, I do not guarantee any particular outcome for your birth. Though studies have shown the overwhelming health, medical, and emotional benefits gained from utilizing a doula during birth, **no doula can guarantee any particular outcome.**

x____

Mother Partner Date

x____

Grateful Life Doula Apprentice Date

Postpartum Doula Agreement: What is my role as a postpartum doula?

I provide physical, emotional, spiritual and educational support any time after your child's birth. I will respect your role as caregiver and decision-maker for your baby, supporting the parenting choices you make. I can help you maintain a calm and peaceful household. I will share my skills and assist with household chores, errands, cooking, and childcare for siblings, as needed and if requested. I will keep our conversations and details about your care confidential unless there is a cause for concern.

Fees

Postpartum doula fees are typically $25-40 per hour, with a six (6) hour minimum. You may prepay for more hours if you prefer. Should you cancel after entering into this agreement, but prior to your 36th week gestation, your fee will be refunded, except for a $50 retainer fee to compensate for my time in blocking out your postpartum hours, which may result in turning away other clients. After 37 weeks, all fees are nonrefundable.

Services

1. I will do one free consultation
2. Prenatal visits at your home (baby care, sibling preparation, child proofing).
3. Continuous physical and emotional support (listening to your birth story, your fears/frustrations/concerns, observing your postpartum recovery).
4. Baby care education and support (assist in bathing, feeding, comforting the baby, cutting baby's nails, organizing the nursery/your home, etc.).
5. Breastfeeding or supplementing support / Preparing nutritious meals
6. Maintaining simple housework (laundry, vacuuming, emptying garbage, straightening up the house, dust, dishes, etc.).
7. Watching the baby and/or older children so Mom/Dad/Partner can rest
8. Referrals to other professionals as needed / Unlimited telephone, text, and email contact
9. I will help with self-care recovery, postpartum comfort measures, infant care, parenting information, and aid with learning to feed and care for the baby.
10. Support could include preparing simple meals and snacks, assisting with light household tasks, and other forms of support as appropriate and necessary.

Limitation of Services

I do NOT perform major house cleaning tasks (ex: washing windows or yard work). I will NOT perform clinical tasks, medical assessments or evaluations nor do I provide medical advice or diagnoses for mother or baby. I am NOT able to provide transportation for mother, baby, or family.

If I am unable to provide any postpartum support due to unpredictable scheduling conflicts, I agree to either find a replacement doula or refund the deposit. In the event of illness, emergency or severe weather, every effort will be made to reschedule services as soon as I am aware that I cannot keep our appointment. Payment for that day will be applied to future service if already paid.

Client: I will communicate my needs to the doula as her duties will depend on my priorities and particular needs that day. I also, hereby give my permission for my doula to write details and share information with the understanding that it is for those working directly with me or my family and for the benefit of our care or data purposes. If I am unable to keep my appointment with my doula, I agree to give the doula at least 24 hours' notice. If I do not, my deposit will NOT be returned to me or applied to fees.

Postpartum Contract

Postpartum Doula Support is $______ per hour. Payment is due at the end of each shift.

Schedule: Mornings Afternoons Evenings Overnights S M T W TH F S Hour

Services are expected to begin around (date) _____________and continue until_____________.

Due Date: _____________ Deposit: $________ Fee: $________/Hr.

Signatures

x____

Client's Signature Date

x____Grateful

Life Doula Signature Date

Grateful Life Doula Services: Evaluation for Co-laboring Birth Support

Mother's Name____

Baby's DOB_____________ Location__________________________

Doula's Name____

1.) Was the doula professional in her conduct with you/partner and staff?
   Y N

2.) Were the techniques and comfort measures helpful to you?
   Y N

3.) Did she give information, suggestions and provide advocacy?
   Y N

4.) Was the emotional/ spiritual support a benefit to you/partner/ family/friends?
   Y N

5.) Would you recommend having a doula to someone else?
   Y N

Rate each category, so we can improve our services and offer the best care.

Evaluation:	Excellent	Good	Fair	Poor
	1	2	3	4

Professional _____ Physical _____ Emotional _____ Spiritual _____

Any other comments or suggestions?

Consent to Ministry Form

I voluntarily consent to be ministered by____________________________.

I understand that the facilitator I am seeing today is not a licensed counselor or professional Psychologist and there is no guarantee of results. I fully accept this inner healing process and do not hold anyone responsible for any outcome that may surface because of today's meeting or at any further time in the future.

I am not legally bound to continue this path if I choose to stop at any time during the process, however, I realize there might be barriers or delays with my ability to experience complete healing, deliverance, or freedom if I do so. My intention is to partner with the people I am walking on this journey with and finish this process to completion. I understand that there will likely be a time of aftercare and follow-up to empower, equip and encourage me to remain connected with the truth I have received.

Participant:____

Date:_____________

Facilitator:____

Date:_____________

Group Guidelines:

1. **Relationship**—Relationships are built on trust, therefore what is shared is to be confidential. Our hope is that each one will feel secure in knowing that the words they say will be a benefit and will not be repeated to anyone else.
2. **Respect**—We will be respectful of others by allowing everyone the opportunity to share. Feel free to ask questions and learn.
3. **Reflection—**Reflection is allowing the light of truth to become transparent to others. Unity is strengthened when we are open and accountable to each other in love.

REFERENCES

After praise and encouragement: Emotional support strategies used by birth doulas in the USA and Canada. Midwifery, Sept. 16. Gruber, K.J. et al. (2013)

Anatomy, Physiology and Philosophy of Breastfeeding. Retrieved August, 2016 from http://fhs.mcmaster.ca/surgery/documents/ap_breastfeed.pdf

Bible Gateway. Retrieved August, 2016 from https://www.biblegateway.com/passage/

Birth Trauma: Definition and Statistics Penny Simkin, PT, PATTCh Founder 2015 http://pattch.org/resource-guide/traumatic-births-and-ptsd-definition-and-statistics/

Brewer, S. MD., Bhattacharya, S., Davies, J. MD., Meredith, S. MD., & Preston, P. MD. (2011). *The pregnant body book* (Dr. P. Moran, Ed.). New York, NY: DK Publishing

Can a Difficult Birth Create Psychological Problems Later? Lorri Craig 2015 http://lorricraig.com/psychologist/general-psychology/difficult-birth-psychological-problems/

ChartsBin Statistics Collector Team. (2011). Capital punishment around the world. Retrieved from http://chartsbin.com/view/1182

Childbirth Connection. "Best Evidence: Labor Support." 2011. Retrieved on 3/17/2012 from http://www.childbirthconnection.org/article.asp?ck=10174&ClickedLink= 257&area=27 Eftekhary, S. et al. (2010)

Cleansing Stream Notebook. (2004). Van Nuys, CA: Cleansing Stream Ministries.

Comfort measures during labor and delivery: Non-pharmacologic methods. Retrieved 2016, August http://www.nwh.org/community-health-resources/maternity-guide/labor-and-delivery/comfort-measures-non-pharma/

Continuous support for women during childbirth. Cochrane Database of Systematic Reviews, Issue 2. Hodnett, E.D., et al. (2012); Issue 10. Art. No.: CD003766. Hunter, C. (2012)

Crisis Care Network- info@crisiscare.com

DONA International (2001). *Dads, partners and doulas: Key players on mother's labor support team.* [Topic Sheet]. Retrieved from http://www.dona.org/PDF/DadsandDoulas.pdf

"Going Beyond the Call of Doula": A grounded theory analysis of the diverse roles community-based doulas play in the lives of pregnant and parenting adolescent mothers. Journal of Perinatal Education, 19(4): 24- 40. Gilliland, A.L. (2010)

Doula care, birth outcomes and costs among Medicaid beneficiaries. American Journal of Public Health, Apr 103(4): 113-21.

Evaluation of student-nurse doula program: an analysis of doula interventions and their impact on labor analgesia and cesarean birth. Journal of Midwifery and Womens Health, 57(1): 28-34. Smith, L. (2010)

Fathers suffer PTSD following traumatic childbirth experience. Janel Shorthouse. October, 2014

http://www.abc.net.au/local/photos/2014/10/14/4106590.htm
FocusOnTheFamily.com

Green, Michael. MD. (2012, June 4). *Dilation, effacement, station.* Retrieved from http://medtwice.com/dilation-effacement-station/

Harms, R. W., MD. (Ed.). (2004). *Mayo clinic guide to a healthy pregnancy.* New York, NY: HarperCollins Publishers Inc.

Help for Doulas Who Are Traumatized by Births They Attend
Penny Simkin, PT, CD(DONA) International Doula Volume 23, Issue 1 2015

How Your Breasts Make Milk: The Physiology of Breastfeeding
Retrieved August, 2016 from http://www.ameda.com/breastfeeding/anatomy-physiology

Hybels, B. (2009). *Courageous leadership.* United States of America: Zondervan
http://www.doulas.info/publi/pro/200605-JOGNNjournalmag.pdf

https://c.ymcdn.com/sites/www.awhonn.org/resource/resmgr/Downloadables/perinatalqualitymeasures_ref.pdf

http://www.jognn.org/article/S0884-2175(15)30584-0/pdf
https://course.trainingdoulas.com/wp-content/uploads/2016/01/physioloigical-birth-consensus-statement-final-may-18-2012-final.pdf

ICEA Doula Training Guide, 2013. Paterno, M.T. et al. (2012)

International Childbirth Education Association 2501 Aerial Center Pkwy Ste. 103, Morrisville, NC 27560 • Phone 919-863-9487 • Fax 919-459-2075• www.icea.org

Impact of doulas on healthy birth outcomes. Journal of Perinatal Education, 22(1): 49-58. Hodnett, E.J. et al. (2011)

Intimate space within institutionalized birth: women's experiences birthing with doulas. Anthropological Medicine, 19(3): 315-26. Klaus, M.H.; Kennell, J.H.; Klaus, P.H.

LaFavor, J. & Pixley, J. (2012) *Heart of a doula* [DVD]. United States: Embracing Miracles Ministries.

LaFavor, J. & Pixley, J. (2012). *Making Disciples*. Dallas, TX: Creative Press

Lambert, T. (n.d.). *A brief history of punishments*. Retrieved from http://www.localhistories.org/pun.html

Maltby, L. E., & Hall, T. W. (2012). Trauma, attachment, and spirituality: A case study Midwives' and doulas' perspectives on the role of the doula in Australia: a qualitative study, Midwifery, 27(4): 509-16

Miaese, M. (June, 2004). *Human rights protection.* Retrieved from http://www.beyondintractability.org/essay/human-rights-protect

Milton, Sarah H. MD. (2016, February 25). *Normal labor and delivery.*

(Isaacs, Christine, MD., Ed.). Retrieved from

http://emedicine.medscape.com/article/260036-overview

Montaldo, Charles. (July, 2015). *What is the crime of murder?* Retrieved from http://crime.about.com/od/Crime_101/f/What-Is-Murder.htm

Mothering the Mother: How a doula can help you have a shorter, easier and healthier birth. Addison Wesley Publishing Company. 1993. Updated in 2002 and renamed The Doula Book: How a trained labor companion can help you have a shorter, easier and healthier birth. Perseus Books Group. Kozhimannil, K.B., et al. (2013)

Remer, Molly. (2008, February 4). Good Foods to Eat in Labor [Web log post]. Retrieved from https://talkbirth.me/2008/02/04/good-foods-to-eat-in-labor/http://www.mayoclinic.org/healthy-lifes/fitness/tylein-depth/exercise/

Research and Clinical Studies
https://www.bellybelly.com.au/birth/birth-rituals-around-the-world/
https://evidencebasedbirth.com/the-evidence-for-doulas/
https://www.dona.org/what-is-a-doula/benefits-of-a-doula/
https://www.npr.org/sections/health- shots/2016/01/15/463223250/doula-support-for-pregnant-women-could-improve-care-reduce-costs
https://www.ncbi.nlm.nih.gov/pmc/articles/PMC3647727/
https://nmaahc.si.edu/explore/stories/historical-significance-doulas-and-midwives
https://teachinghistory.org
Smith, Stephen. (Ed.). (2016, August 18). Retrieved from https://www.openbible.info/topics/the_body_of_christ

Sprinkle, J. (2006a). *Biblical law and its relevance.* Lanham, MD: University of America

Sprinkle, J. (2015b). *Leviticus and numbers* (M. Strauss & J. Walton, Eds.). Grand Rapids, MI: Baker Publishing Group

St. Louis, Catherine. (2013, July 10). Study finds benefits in delaying severing of umbilical cord. *New York Times*. Retrieved from http://www.nytimes.com/2013/07/11/health/study-endorses-later-severing-of-umbilical-cord.html

Teen Pregnancy: Facts

a. Pregnancy
| October 2001By: Isabel V. Sawhill
http://www.brookings.edu/research/papers/2001/10/childrenfamilies-sawhill

b. Abortion/ Miscarriage
Linda Lowen Women's Issues Expert
http://womensissues.about.com/od/datingandsex/tp/Teenpregancy.htm

c. Adoption
http://www.americanadoptions.com/pregnant/adoption-questions

- Race-(KathrynKostandStanleyHenshaw2014 http://www.guttmacher.org/pubs/USTPtrends10.pdf).

The Impact of Birthing Practices on Breastfeeding, 2nd Edition. Jones and Bartlett Publishers. Stevens, J. et al. (2011)

The life of a Canadian doula: successes, confusion and conflict. Journal of Obstetrics and Gynecology Canada, 32(7): 642-9. Gentry, Q.M. et al. (2010)

University of Washington Medical Center (2004, December). *Perinatal Education Program/Maternal and Infant Care Clinic Checklist of Comfort Measures for Labor*. Retrieved from http://www.uwmedicine.org/services/obstetrics/documents/Comfort-Measures-For-Labor.pdf

Traumahealinginstitute.org /Traumahealingbasics.org

Varnum, P. & Ham, K. (2006). *Fearfully and wonderfully made* [DVD]. United States: Answers in Genesis

Vieth, V (2012). What would walther do? Applying law and gospel to victims and perpetrators of child sexual abuse. *Journal of Psychology & Theology 40*(4), 257-273.

Wenham, J. G. (2008). *Numbers: An introduction and commentary.* Downers Grove, IL: InterVarsity Press

World Health Organization. (2009). *The physiological basis of breastfeeding.* Retrieved by http://www.ncbi.nlm.nih.gov/books/NBK148970/

Zimmerman, G.H. (2013, July). Birth trauma: Posttraumatic stress disorder after childbirth. *International Journal of Childbirth Education. 28*(3), 61-66

ABOUT THE AUTHOR

Jessica LaFavor CD (DONA) is a dedicated mother of three grown children and a Mimi (Grandma) of one. She is the founder of Grateful Life Ministries, LLC, and manager of a wellness and beauty e-commerce store, Grateful Life Retail- keeping families healthy, growing, and full of love! https://www.amway.com/myshop/GratefulLifeRetail.

She is the Vice President of Embracing Miracles, a certified doula, a peer recovery specialist, and a trauma healing facilitator. Along with that, she has been a trained prayer minister, a keynote conference speaker, and a published author. She is the Women's Director of Next Chapter Ministries in Rochester, MN, serving those impacted by the cycle of incarceration. She has been an advocate in areas such as trauma, addiction/recovery, homelessness, and mental health.

Her 25+ years' experience in the doula field includes certification through *DONA International* as a birth doula, providing childbirth education, having postpartum doula training by *ProDoula*, and conducting "Heart of a Doula" workshops for various groups and organizations. Her favorite Bible verse is Psalm 119:2, "Blessed are they that keep the testimonies of the Lord with their whole heart." Jessica was born with a hole in her heart and has a miraculous testimony of how God made her heart whole!

The Grateful Life team hosted *Women of Strength* events for 10 years as Jessica served as the co-pastor at the Church of the Nazarene in Kasson, MN. She co-authored a children's ministry curriculum called, "Making Disciples." She was a part of the development team and taught at the Train a Child Center (TACC). Her passion is to equip and train others for community leadership. Her heart is legacy— to make an impact on the next generation.

Grateful Life Ministries

To contact Jessica, go to or call:

gratefullifeministries@gmail.com

507-271-4784

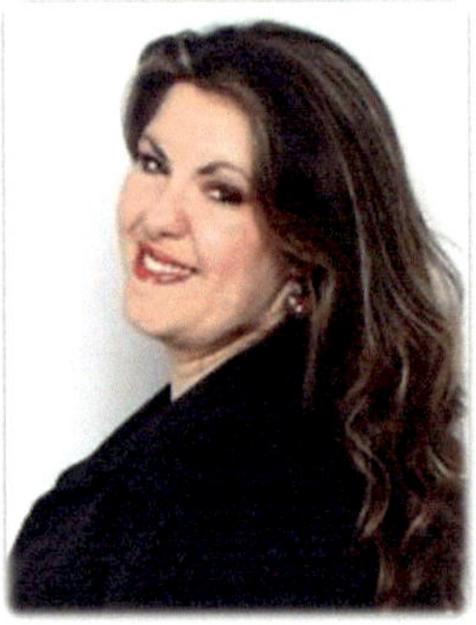

Made in the USA
Las Vegas, NV
03 November 2026

57421803R00100